Praise for *Get a*

'Clever, kind, funny and wise, this book is an uplifting
and useful addition to your self-help library. Kate's
voice is such a big, positive part of the evolving
mental health conversation.'
Daisy Buchanan, *How to Be a Grown-Up*

'In her wittily titled no-nonsense guide to mental
health, [Kate] writes about her experiences of
depression with insight, honesty and even humour.'
Independent

'A quirky, candid memoir... This will have
huge appeal to anyone who feels they're at rock
bottom; it will also enlighten their friends.'
Evening Standard

'Refreshingly irreverent... [Kate] strikes the perfect
balance between being light-hearted but still gritty, honest
and very real. For anyone experiencing depression,
this book will help you feel seen and understood. It
will help you advocate for yourself, and break the
inertia with tonics you feel genuinely moved to try. It's also
a compassionate guide for those supporting loved ones.'
Suzy Reading, Author and Psychologist

'A raw, honest, necessarily uncomfortable
and funny insight into depression.'
Jo Usmar, *This Book Will Make You Happy*

Kate Lucey is an experienced digital journalist, public speaker, and panel mediator and has worked with brands from *Cosmopolitan* to *Sunday Times Style* to advise on how to effectively talk to millennials. She regularly writes about mental health for a range of publications and is currently living in Paris. *Get a Grip, Love* is her first book.

GET A GRIP, LOVE

Kate Lucey

HQ

ONE PLACE. MANY STORIES

AUTHOR'S NOTE:
Some names have been changed to protect the privacy of individuals.

HQ
An imprint of HarperCollins*Publishers* Ltd
1 London Bridge Street
London SE1 9GF

www.harpercollins.co.uk

HarperCollins Publishers
Macken House, 39/40 Mayor Street Upper,
Dublin 1 D01 C9W8, Ireland

This edition 2023

1
First published in Great Britain by
HQ, an imprint of HarperCollins*Publishers* Ltd 2021

Copyright © Kate Lucey 2021

Kate Lucey asserts the moral right to be identified as the author of this work.
A catalogue record for this book is available from the British Library.

ISBN: 978-0-00-840108-5

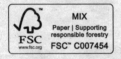

This book is produced from independently certified FSC™ paper
to ensure responsible forest management.

For more information visit: www.harpercollins.co.uk/green

This book is set in 11.7/16 pt. Sabon by Type-it As, Norway

Printed and Bound in the UK using 100% Renewable Electricity at
CPI Group (UK) Ltd, Croydon, CR0 4YY

To anyone who's ever sat in their misery and
not been able to see a way out of it.

Also to me, without whom this book
would not have been possible.

Contents

Foreword

I would bet my life that there is nobody, nobody, who will come out of this pandemic and be exactly the same as when they went in. We watched a war unfold around us. Nobody will be unscathed.

Sorry to start this chapter off with total doom, but those words from psychotherapist Claire Goodwin-Fee pretty much sum it all up, don't they?

At the time of writing, we are halfway through year three of this plague. What we thought would be over within a few months has lasted longer than it took to build the Eiffel Tower (two years, two months and five days), and the amount of time Bill Cosby spent in prison (just under three years) and might just last longer than Elton John's Farewell Tour (four years, ten months). If this thing outlives Liza Minnelli I swear to God...

When lockdowns were first announced, it all seemed like a fun bit of novelty, didn't it? A big global sleepover. All the pressure was off, we didn't have any obligations to go out and socialise, ALL the plans were cancelled and we were free to sludge around our homes and binge-watch reality shows about Australians cheating on each other.

We had group video calls and downloaded new apps so we could play games with our pals. We attended endless quizzes and games nights. My family did a sodding Murder Mystery for which we all dressed up in costumes and put on accents, for chrissakes. We made banana bread. We clapped for the NHS. We stepped up our WhatsApp groups and we sent never-ending memes about Joe Exotic. It was actually pretty fun!

Until it wasn't.

As the lockdown wore on and the virus started to really get its claws in, the previously novel 'locky-dee' very much became 'horrific state-sanctioned isolation', which, combined with news and notifications about daily death tolls and Italian doctors not being able to treat anyone over the age of sixty because they were so overwhelmed with patients and deaths... well... it got a bit much, didn't it? The virus was spreading rapidly around the world and all we could do was sit and watch, and hope it didn't sink its teeth into someone we loved.

Turns out that living in a permanent state of anxiety is not so hot for our collective wellbeing. The pandemic and everything that came along with it (political sprawls, anti-vaxxers, redundancies, poverty, domestic violence and a feeling of never-ending hopelessness...) triggered mental health issues for so many. In the first year of the Covid-19 pandemic, global prevalence of anxiety and depression increased by a massive 25 per cent, according to a scientific brief released by the World Health Organization (WHO).[1]

Medical journal *The Lancet* published a study into the effects of the pandemic on global mental health, in which they estimated that Miss 'Rona had brought on approximately 53 million additional cases of major depressive disorder. It's hard to imagine 53 million, but it's essentially the same as the *whole of Spain* getting cursed with depression (though if this did happen, it would be called *depresión masiva,* which is entirely sexier).

Of course, while many of these 53 million new cases would have been people just like me – enduring being stuck indoors for more of the same every day with spiralling thoughts, and boredom that led to some really questionable TV choices – it also includes many of those who were quite literally on the frontline of the pandemic. Our medical professionals.

Hospitals called on all available medical staff to help attend the Covid wards at the pandemic's peak. Many of these medics hadn't thought about a lung for decades as they were busy specialising in other areas, and so were likely pretty terrified to go into work after receiving their one-day refresher course and being told to suit up as if they were going to war. Doctors who'd worked as breast cancer surgeons for years were left feeling like the work experience kids when they didn't really know how to work a ventilator. I've been told in confidence that some quite physically hid, for fear that they might kill someone due to their lack of respiratory knowledge.

I can only imagine the effect that this pressure must have had on their mental health. (Can I take this moment to say hello to anyone who worked on the frontline during the height of the pandemic and is now here because their brain got dark as a result? You are a hero and I wish I could give each and every one of you an enormous hug and a really good sandwich with posh condiments and really good chips.)

In the UK more than 27,000 members of the NHS left their jobs between the first two waves of coronavirus. The highest number of resignations on record. And who can blame them?

The deteriorating mental health of those working for the NHS prompted Claire, the incredible psychotherapist whose quote opens this chapter, to launch a not-for-profit business that provided mental health support to those working on the frontlines. Claire told me that one nurse she was speaking to eventually quit after sixteen years and went to work at McDonald's, justifying the move with the stone cold facts that 'it's about the same salary and I don't have to pay to park my car'.

This isn't to say, at all, that you should sit up, chin up, tits out and get yourself together because you 'didn't have it as bad as the doctors', or 'at least my family are alive' or 'I got to rewatch *The Twilight Saga*'. Those flippant suggestions are EXACTLY what this book is not about. Or are they exactly what this book *is* about, in as much as it slags them off?

Actually, yes, these off-hand, trashy suggestions are the exact motivation behind this book. These pages will call out the trope of unhelpful comments; over the course of these chapters, you're going to realize that this really isn't a competition to see who has experienced the biggest trauma. When it comes to the pandemic, we all need to take in the fact that we went through something that changed us, no matter how trivial it may seem compared to those on the frontline. If your brain is telling you to pull yourself together because 'at least you didn't have it as bad as other people did', then it's time to tell your brain to hush up. We all experienced things that were stressors, aggressors and downers. Just because you weren't developing a vaccine or working in the hospital wards, doesn't mean it didn't suck. As Claire cheerfully put it, 'I do think that we will all have some level of trauma within ourselves because of it.'

The fact is that the pandemic caused many people immeasurable trauma. And, when you consider Maslow's hierarchy of needs, it's easy to see why. Abraham Maslow was a psychologist who came up with the theory that every human has a hierarchy of psychological needs. As in, there are things we all need in our lives in order not to be a mess. The theory is that if we can have each need fulfilled, we'll be functioning and admirable and have really shiny hair.

The needs are generally displayed in a triangle diagram, which really is a pretty apt little pyramid depicting what we all allegedly need to feel motivated to live life: safety, love and belonging, and self-esteem. For a lot of us, the pandemic stripped away every single one of these needs, so it's no wonder we felt shite.

One of the most basic needs outlined in the theory (at the bottom of the pyramid) is the need for safety and security. Well, that was removed pretty damn swiftly when the news broke that we could, at any moment, catch a virus that could kill us but would more likely kill the people we loved. So chill! We can't see the virus, touch it or smell it, and in the early days we couldn't test for it. But good luck, yeah? When I was feeling like I was putting others in danger and there was nothing I could do to control it, I absolutely started to feel like a mess, and the cartoon raincloud over my head began to grow and darken.

Another need deemed essential (and another level up in the jazzy triangle) is the need for love and belonging. I mean, I don't know about you, but the lack of touch was what got me in the end. As someone who is quite overly 'huggy', and would absolutely be described as 'touchy-feely' (not in a Weinstein way, just to confirm), I didn't realize how much I actually needed affection and human touch. I spent the first lockdown on my own in a small apartment in Paris, and while the boulangeries were deemed essential businesses (honestly, thank fuck for that), hugs and touching were verging on being akin to murder.

Turns out that my needy-need to be hugged is an Actual Thing, and there's an official name for that longing for physical contact: Skin Hunger. EXCUSE ME? HOW ABSOLUTELY GROSS IS THAT? But it's true, alas. Dr Kitty Wheate, a medical anthropologist, wrote about Skin Hunger during lockdown for the University of Edinburgh, saying that even people who live with and have access to hugs from people they love can struggle with it, because 'life may simply be so tough right now that your need for connection and comfort feels ravenous'. Which certainly goes some way to explaining my constant need to be fondled all the time: because I'm WELL SAD.

So, yes, while being isolated from other people initially may have felt a little freeing, it eventually started to get fairly bleak.

Towards the top of Maslow's emotional Toblerone is the need for self-esteem. Ah yes, self-respect... wonder what that feels like. I, like many, was made redundant at the start of the pandemic, mid-way through the first lockdown (#girlboss!). For so many of us who were out of work due to redundancy or being put on furlough, the days locked indoors lost all sense of structure and purpose. Being out of work, even temporarily, has a huge impact on our self-esteem, self-respect and feelings of accomplishment – and worrying about money isn't exactly a welcome new way to spend time. Days went by where I achieved nothing apart from setting a new record for vodka imbibing. Having nowhere to go and nothing required of me to do ended up propelling me into unhealthy habits, rather than encouraging me to learn French and take up cross-stitching in between working on my abs, as everyone else seemed to be doing.

I don't know about you, but thinking I was 'rocking at life' because I was having a joint, a cocktail and watching *Will & Grace* at 3 p.m. on a Tuesday took quite a quick, steep plummet into making me feel like a feral wretch who was gaining weight and generally being a waste of human life.

We went through something humans are *not designed to do*, and the result of that was pretty catastrophic on our minds, regardless of whether we were fighting on the frontline or not.

I was personally delighted at the start of the pandemic: my fake jazz hands were put away and my fake happy mask was taken off. My forced coat-hanger smile was removed, and any attempts at maintaining a Positive Mental Attitude were put to an absolute halt. There was no need to pretend to be a happy, 'normal', functioning person – which is all pretty damn exhausting for someone with depression. I could wash off all the pretences and just be fucking sad if I didn't have the energy to pretend otherwise. Besides the video calls, I could fester in my little hut of darkness and silence. Finally. Perhaps this would be the sweet release my dark soul had always needed?

Not so much. Before long, I started to feel supremely stupid for not knowing how good I actually had it in the Before Times, when I could go outside and sit in cafés or see live music or hug a friend and squeeze them so tightly that my love for them would surely transfer into their body through osmosis, or something. And I know that I'm not the only one.

The chunkiest part of the pandemic might (hopefully please, gawwwd) be behind us, but the trauma of having these needs stripped from us for so long is only just sinking in for many. Everyone lost the ability to live a normal, functioning life, and according to Maslow, we had everything we needed to be psychologically stable completely taken away.

And that's not all. Huge numbers of families of patients on the Covid wards were robbed of any gradual emotional build-up towards the death of a loved one, which left them with raw shock. Conversations that would have usually been had in person, in the hospital, after a phone call asking someone to physically come to the hospital, just happened on the phone with no warning. While it's pretty gloomy to think about, it's likely that we'll still be trying to muddle our way through this unresolved trauma in the years to come. Living through notable moments in history sucks.

Licensed psychologist Seth J. Gillihann, PhD and author of *Mindful Cognitive Behavioral Therapy* (YEAH, he's legit), has some advice for those who find themselves in this situation:

I would encourage them, as I would anyone who's bereaved, to make space for their grief, and for the unpredictability and just messiness of it. It's not a linear or stepwise process. It's more surprising and unpredictable than we expect. There's no 'wrong or right' way to do this, so allow yourself to release expectations or judgments about what you 'should' be feeling or doing. Challenge any thoughts (or others' suggestions) that you 'should be further along,' or that you 'need to express your emotions,' etc. Grief is different for everyone.

Let go of questions about whether you're 'doing this right.' Trust yourself. There is a wisdom in you that knows how to grieve, even if it feels like you have no idea what you're doing. That's OK. You don't have to know. Just stay close to your experience and keep making room for all of it.

Even those who haven't lost a loved one might find themselves suffering from confusion, trembling or debilitating nightmares, which are common symptoms of post-Traumatic stress disorder (PTSD). PTSD was originally called 'shell shock', when a psychologist noticed all of those symptoms in soldiers who had survived World War One. Now we use PTSD to refer to trauma that occurs at least a month after a traumatic event. Claire told me:

> *The deeper and more significant trauma is coming out now because it has the space to expand. The pandemic has gone on for so long that more people are being diagnosed with CPTSD, which is <u>complex</u> PTSD, related to ongoing trauma rather than attached to one time. When you're emotionally injured from something, it will eventually come out in a physical sense.*

Did you hear that? The effects of the pandemic have literally caused people to suffer with CPTSD. And yet, even now, a lot of us are trying to buckle-up and soldier on, and not really take into account what the pandemic did to us all. We have been *through* it. In fact, if you feel like you're still the person you were in the long gay summer of 2019 then I personally am very suspicious of you. Feeling overwhelmed, exhausted and drained doesn't mean that you're weak or can't cope. It means that you're human.

There aren't any concrete details around the number of people diagnosed with pandemic-related PTSD, but the *Psychiatric Times* (sounds like a fun place to work) says that it's most commonly felt by a few specific groups of people – which actually probably account for a hefty percentage of the population:

> *Different groups have met the qualifying criteria for post-traumatic stress disorder (PTSD) according to DSM-5 as a result of the pandemic: those who have themselves suffered from serious Covid-19 illness and potential death; individuals who, as family members and health care workers, have witnessed others' suffering and death; individuals who have learned about the death or risk of death of a family member or friend due to the virus; and individuals who have experienced extreme exposure to aversive details (e.g. journalists, first responders, medical examiners, and hospital personnel).*[2]

While I've certainly experienced traumatic events (being sexually assaulted, being bullied at work, being stalked and gaslit by an angry man, missing out on front-row tickets to Boyzone in 1997…), I don't consider myself to have PTSD. This isn't because I'm 'stronger' than those who do, or that my circumstances 'weren't actually that bad, love', it's just because our brains react differently to life and all its unpleasant surprises. Even what could be considered the same experience can be completely different to different people.

Symptoms of PTSD tend to include any of the fun little devils below:

- Finding yourself constantly re-living the traumatic event. This could be through nightmares, or through vivid daydreams that don't feel like recalling memories, but instead feel like you're going through it all over again.

- Becoming upset when you encounter anything that reminds you of the event, and going out of your way to avoid anything that might make you think of it.
- Generally being more emotional than usual and feeling like you can't handle your feelings or manage your responses to things.
- Feeling like the world is no longer safe, and catastrophising the worst possible outcomes from every event (this is also a symptom of generalised anxiety disorder).
- Hyperreactivity, which is finding yourself startled at loud noises, pained by bright lights and generally anxious and panicked when there are noise interruptions around you.
- Being in a cage of rage. It's common for people going through PTSD to be highly irritable, prone to angry outbursts and behaving in a recklessly self-destructive manner. This can also be a symptom of bipolar disorder, if it also occurs alongside periods of elation, extreme joy and happiness and spontaneous decision making and actions.

So, what if you find yourself saying 'yup, yes, oh definitely' to that list of symptoms and realising that you're living with PTSD when you thought you just needed to pull yourself together and get a grip? (Hi, book title! Yep, this book is entirely against that school of thinking and is full of the tools and tips you need to realize that you do NOT need to get a grip, love. So strap in!)

The best advice is to talk to a professional medical practitioner. Like with all mental health illnesses, everyone's traumatic experiences are profoundly different, and it may be medication, counselling, or a combination of both that make the biggest positive difference to you.

If I could be so bold as to put a PoSiTiVe SpIn on things, though, I think we've all cottoned on to some valuable intel about ourselves over the course of the pandemic. Yes, the pandemic was shit. People died who perhaps wouldn't have if everyone had been able to wear their masks and stay away from each other from the beginning. We were starved of our loved ones while politicians had mad wine and cheese raves. We thought we might kill our grans. We couldn't go to funerals. Nobody could dance. Wait… what was the positive point I was going to make? I'm sure I had one…

Oh yes, well, it turns out that life wasn't so great in the first place, and for a lot of us it took being locked down to realize that we needed to make some changes to how we go about our lives. I wasn't alone in thinking that lockdown was going to be a brilliant couple of weeks of alone time and no enforced fun – which is pretty wild anyway, when you think about it. I asked how other people felt when lockdowns were first announced in their countries, and the general feeling – even among those without depression – seemed to be, 'Oh YES, thank crap for this, everyone will leave me alone.'

Here are some of the responses I got:

- 'The biggest emotion I felt when the lockdown was announced was relief. It felt like an opportunity to live life at the pace I wanted to. To be insular and anonymous and not be judged for that. To wake up and not worry about what the day might bring, who I might encounter and whether my depression and social anxiety could handle that.'
- 'I've always felt the pressure to make believable excuses when I didn't want to see friends, rather than just saying

no. So being able to say, "Ahh bloody Covid stopping our plans!" was great. It was a huge relief.'

- 'I had a baby during lockdown, and it was actually pretty perfect. The number of visitors people get when they have a new baby is crazy, but nobody was allowed to come over. I didn't have to get out of my PJs or try to look respectable or like I had myself together.'
- 'Lockdown felt like a get-out-of-jail-free card for all those social occasions I didn't want to attend, yet previously felt I had to for fear of not *living*.'
- 'I had absolutely zero FOMO for the first time in my life. I knew I wasn't missing out on anything, and that the place I needed to be was exactly where I was.'

It does make you wonder if before we went into lockdown we were all just living lives of vicious lies. Were we all just tolerating each other while wishing we were at home making a dent on the sofa? Were we all too scared to say no to things we didn't want to do?

Essentially, yes.

I'm definitely not the only one who said yes to invitations because I didn't want to let people down. Who said yes to having visitors all the time because I didn't want to be rude, or who stayed late at work because I felt like I needed to put more effort in, rather than having a chat about unrealistic workloads. In fact, Claire said to me:

I think we really were quite unhealthy pre-pandemic. I mean, look at all these people who've quit their jobs! The Great Resignation happened, and everyone wanted to change their lives and the way that they work.

Indeed, when all other distractions were removed and we were locked in our homes with only our work to focus on, a lot of us realized that we hated our jobs, or couldn't stomach our managers any longer. More than 40 million people left their jobs during the pandemic – not because they were fed up with earning money, but because they were fed up with the conditions in which they were expected to do it.[3]

I think this is brilliant; so many more of us are now standing up to demand humane treatment at work. Flexible hours. Remote working. No commutes. Better pay and benefits. The majority of people who left their jobs were in retail or hospitality, customer-facing industries famous for unreliable hours, shoddy pay and shoddy treatment by the public – none of which contribute to a serene and glistening mental state. If being put on furlough seemed like a gift, going back to work was a hellscape.

Even now I'm still noticing a new trend of friends and colleagues tolerating less, people-pleasing less, and knowing their worth, and it feels like I'm joining them and putting myself and my mental health first. Where we used to be loyal to bosses and companies, we're now starting to be loyal to our mental wellbeing. If employees are being treated patronisingly by a manager, they know that a manager elsewhere will give them respect, and so they'll quit. If they're not being offered benefits, they'll negotiate a higher salary. If their job is thankless, they'll go find one that isn't. I love the drama.

After wanging on about my mental health in a book, I'm a lot more comfortable talking about it out loud to other humans (and my sister's cat). This probably sounds obvious, but it took a while. It's really much easier to write things down than it is to look someone in the eye and say things to them. If I'm in a depression funk (truly the most un-funky of funks) I won't make up an excuse for staying in, I'll tell the truth. Often, whoever I'm talking to will offer some support, a chat or some ice cream, and remind me that I'm loved. Assurance, love, comforting chats and ice cream don't come to you if you pretend you've got the shits.

While being locked in with nothing but my own mind for company was horrific, it also allowed me to feel my feelings, all the time, and cry, all the time. While I don't know if this was a good thing or a bad thing, not having to pretend and just being able to exhale and allow the tears to trickle down was a similar relief to that of taking your bra off at the end of the day. This was also the first time I'd ever lived alone, and it felt like I was finally able to truly be myself in my own space – and reader, my true self is pretty gross.

Now, whenever I speak to people who tell me that they're feeling sad and trying not to feel that way, I advise them to absolutely allow themselves to feel that way: to have a cry and let it out. Pretending that you're not sad is knackering, and sometimes having a cry and just feeling the feelings can be pretty powerfully helpful. I think that crying is sometimes like the feeling you get when you know you need to sneeze, but it's teasing you for a while and then BAM, ACHOO, OH GOD, THAT FEELS BETTER.

Freud reckoned that crying served an 'intra-individual' purpose of self-soothing, and that following a good ol' sob sesh, said-sobber would be treated to some stress reduction and mood enhancement. It can even (allegedly, according to science) release endorphins. Lucey (that's me) is not so sure about that, but sometimes it can't be helped, and it feels better to just be able to let it out. Like a wee.

The importance of crying more wasn't my only learning during the pandemic; I also discovered what made me happy or tired. Oh, ROUND OF APPLAUSE. Yeah, this seems like a fairly basic learning, but collectively we weren't very good at acknowledging what made us feel these things before Covid kicked off. We now really, *really* know which people we actually give a shit about and want to spend time with – pre-panny we said yes to everything and everyone and hated it. We worked late in the office and missed out on seeing friends. We were glued to our phones. Now we actually want to see each other AND, AAAAND, I truly believe it's made everyone a lot more open and comfortable talking about their mental health. It's also made me personally a lot more relaxed about saying 'no' to invitations from people who I realized I find very draining. Not feeling obliged to please people who make me feel bad about myself, and not feeling rude for rebutting suggestions that people 'pop over and stay for a long weekend'. We all went through shit, together, around the world. A lot of us are still going through it, and we've got a gorgeous collective horrific experience of hell to share. We also learned that sometimes we really do need to be left the fuck alone.

So how do we take these learnings and move forward? And for those of us who picked up a new diagnosis that had been caused by the pandemic – will that shiny new depression go away now that things have returned to 'normal'?

Seth the Psychologist (who I quoted earlier on in this chapter) tells me that:

For most of us, thankfully, pandemic-induced depression will fade as we start doing the things that keep us feeling alive and engaged. It won't be immediate, but it doesn't have to take a long time once we get back to rewarding activities.

Many of us will need to be deliberate about breaking the habit of isolation, which for many will mean pushing through a bit of social anxiety from lack of practice being around others. Depression also saps our interest in doing things – even stuff we enjoy – so we'll probably need to push through some avoidance.

Here's what we know tends to work: make a list of things you would find enjoyable – or used to find enjoyable – and gradually add them to your schedule. Start with the easier ones, and work your way up to more challenging ones. Team up with a buddy if that's helpful, someone who can do the activities with you and act as an accountability partner. We know from many research studies that doing activities every day that are enjoyable and important to you is a powerful antidepressant.

I've made a priority out of spending time with my closest pals, even if it's not for a Big Arranged Occasion. We could sit in the same room while we both work from home together. Run errands to IKEA together, or just go for a walk and a chat. The most mundane activities are super low pressure, and I always come out of them feeling good if I've used the opportunity for some friend-time.

On the flipside, there are also plenty of us whose anxiety and depression decided to burst back onto the scene when the pandemic restrictions were slowly lifted, and we were being thrown back into society. Personally my FOMO (fear of missing out) is back in full swing and forcing me out of the house at every opportunity, but I'm trying to work at remembering that taking time for myself is important, that I can't be everywhere at once, and that whatever I'm missing out on is most likely a bit crap anyway. If this is you, remember, you don't *have* to say yes to everything. You can still say no to the things you don't want to do, and 'I'm not up for it/not feeling up to it/would rather skip this one but let me know when you're next around' are all valid reasons to not. 'I would, but I don't want to' also works.

'Don't aim for things you think you *should* do or that others think you should do – focus on those that you're actually interested in,' said Seth – which sounds obvious when someone else says it, but we seemingly let ourselves be led by *should* before we were locked in. He continued:

Because interest [in general] can be so low in depression, you might need to focus on activities that you <u>used</u> to enjoy, even if they don't seem that fun right now. As you get back to life and activity, the fun will follow.

Alongside those of us who just don't want to interact with people again, or who don't want to get dressed or make chit chat, are those people who are very reasonably still worried about catching Covid-19. When we were put into lockdowns and pummelled with news about the deadly virus killing millions (just over six million at the time of writing) of people around the world, our brains' Fight or Flight response was triggered. For the brains that chose 'Flight, thanks', it's really hard to flip that switch off and get back to 'dum dee dumm nothing to see here' normality. Seth's advice is:

Make a systematic plan to do a little each day, and gradually add more as you're able to. Aim for an effort level of about a four or five on a scale of one to ten – enough to gently push yourself, but not so much that it's overwhelming or leaves you so exhausted it's hard to keep going. And remember to give yourself credit for everything you do, even tiny steps that used to be easy for you. Any step forward counts.

The NHS advice is similar, and focuses around not avoiding things entirely – which can seem like the easiest and safest option, but actually just helps to condition ourselves to permanent avoidance. Instead, the advice is to start with small and manageable challenges, such as meeting one person who you love or at least who respects your concerns, and spending time outdoors together. Absolutely no need to go for a group meal at Prezzo. Even without the pandemic tbh.

We all need to be kinder to ourselves and acknowledge that we, and everyone else we speak to or interact with, have had an awful few years, and that our lives will forever be changed as a result of them. Some of us will have experienced trauma and deep loss, but that doesn't necessarily mean that those of us who didn't lose somebody 'had it better'. We've all been traumatised in some way or another, and it's important that we take time to heal, and make 'the new normal' a lifestyle that we wouldn't be relieved to get a break from if we were told to stop.

The clapbacks

So, what do you actually say when someone pops off about the pandemic affecting us all and dismisses your very legit concerns about the state of your brain? Try these:

'Yep, everyone has been *through it*, which means my depression might be easier for you to understand. Remember lockdown sameness doom? It's that. But worse. Please give me some space/a hug/ice cream.'

'We're all probably a little traumatised by the pandemic, actually. We've been through a life-altering event that hopefully we'll never live through again, and it'll be a while before we feel like we've healed from it. How are you doing?'

Introduction

The state of our collective mental wellbeing is firmly in the gutter. Despite 'the mental health conversation' now being louder than ever, there's a vast crapload of nonsense in the 'actual understanding of mental health' chasm. Speaking up about depression or anxiety is still attached to a fear of being given the boot at work, or being seen as a less fun, less capable, less responsible person and much more of a big sad twat. This is despite the fact that mental health diagnoses are increasing – a combo of 'the conversation' helping more of us get treatment, but also an unforgiving job market, stagnant wages, incredibly high rates of loneliness and extreme burnout driving us to ruin. For those who *are* ready to speak about their mental health, everyone and their boss's friend's sister's dog has a 'miracle cure' to throw at them, and it can be very tricky to separate the fact from the fiction.

Spoiler: this is a book about depression, a tricksy little minx that affects everyone differently and is very personal to every body and brain it resides in. So that means it's also a book about me, and maybe you, and people you love who might have depression themselves. It's a guide for people who might be trying to figure out how to be supportive to someone who's trying to direct their mental health demons into some kind of manageable order while all the demons want to do is piss on their joy and make them feel hopeless.

I've been 'officially' depressed (as in, diagnosed) for six years, and have moved from a very intense 'can't get out of bed' stage to a much more palatable 'separating the illness from myself and trying to actually live life' stage. I've experienced everything from bad therapy, bad meds and bad friends, to good therapy and medication, and solutions that actually work. Also, I'm still alive, so that essentially makes me a sadness boffin. The Steve Jobs of constant sobs. The Brad Pitt of feeling shit. The Meryl Streep of dodgy sleep and the Stephen Fry of having a cry. I have learned a lot and experimented with endless alleged 'cures' or 'aids' for mental health, and have been offered unrequested reams of advice about how to 'cure' my depression. I want to share both the tremendous and the twaddle with you in the hopes that you might either feel SEEN, or might be able to help a pal who is also depressed. In this book I talk bluntly and honestly about what has and hasn't worked for me and for others, what deserves to get in the bin and how to respond to trashy comments that suggest that a bath or 'a few days of fasting' will cure you of your actual mental health illness.

As well as offering my own opinions, I've spoken to lots of other people who have or are suffering with mental illness, as well as some qualified experts to help me offer you a guide, reassurance, a big hug and a fact-book that is as informative as possible. The two people who feature predominantly are Peter Klein and Kate Mason. Peter is with Counselling Directory and has experience running the depression and OCD treatment groups at the Priory. He specializes in treating stress, worry, anxiety, psychosis, depression and OCD. Kate Mason is a chartered clinical psychologist and has supported people suffering psychological and emotional distress since 2002. She worked for the NHS for over fifteen years before setting up her own practice, and also previously worked for the Priory Group. They're both very knowledgeable and smart, and their full details are in the appendix if you'd like to know more about them or to get in touch for counselling. Also, here I'd like to shout out to my personal therapist, Marcelle Casingena, who works online and in North London, and who helped me work through a lot of my dark mess.

It's difficult to know how long I'd been unofficially depressed before my diagnosis. Depression is like bad weather; it comes and goes. Sometimes it's really windy and pouring down for weeks – months, even – and then you get a sunny spell. When it's sunny, does that mean all chance of rain is gone? Not so much.

Was I depressed during my teens when I had periods of feeling extremely sad and hopeless, or was I just 'being a teenager' and reacting to the new batch of hormones that were flooding through me? Or were those painful feelings of desperate sadness, which arrived for seemingly no reason at all, not just 'being a teenager' but really the beginnings of the first patches of depression weather?

Maybe depression started at university, or maybe that was just too many nights out and discovering the 'existential gloom hangover'? Did I just miss my family and put too much pressure on myself to live la vida loca in a slightly tragic suburb of North London? It's hard to say, because I never really addressed any sadness during my student partying as serious.

Or was it when I started working full time and was crying on the way home from work most days, or was that me just being a flake who couldn't cope with 'the real world'? We all feel sad and hopeless sometimes, but how often does 'sometimes' have to be for it to be an illness?

All of this really boils down to the question, 'how does depression pick its victims?' Much research has been done and few conclusions have been drawn. Is it genetic? Some evidence suggests 'maybe, but we need more research' (similar to most studies around depression, just to save you some time in your own research). My childhood was blissful, my parents and sister are my best friends, and I have suffered no extreme trauma – but my family does have a history of mental illness. My maternal grandma, Joanna Williams, who had been living with depression that had been exacerbated by the traumatic death of one of her four children, ended her life in 1986 at the age of 52. But does that mean I was always destined to get depression eventually? There's been a lot of research into 'depression genes' and links to family history, but nothing significant has been discovered as of yet.

There are a lot more resources available today for support, treatment and education than there were in the Eighties, but of course people still kill themselves. I have friends who have attempted to, and friends who have, taken their lives by suicide. When someone ends their own life, those left behind can end up wondering what else they could have done to help; if they could have been kinder or more present or helpful. I hope that the experiences documented in this book will help those who are suffering or have suffered, and those who are surviving relatives of people like Joanna, to see that another person's mental health is not their responsibility. You can help and support, sure, but you can't fix it. The only one who can do that is the individual.

Trying to pin your depression on a 'cause' or a 'reason' is futile. You'd be better off spending your time trying to figure out why

Danny and Sandy flew a sodding car into the sky at the end of *Grease*. Depression can happen to anyone. Sometimes it can be triggered by something traumatic, sometimes it can be based on a lot of heavy self-loathing, sometimes it can be hereditary, and often it just attaches itself to your brain and messes with you for no reason at all. Such fun.

Before I was diagnosed with depression, I would find myself coming home from work and going straight to bed. I would ignore my then-boyfriend in favour of lying in the dark and having a cry, and then feeling guilty for not being able to cope with life. I put it down to the working world being too much for a little snowflake like me, and my boyfriend assumed I was being a cranky cow. I was feeling nothing but darkness on the inside. On the outside, though, I was still functioning 'as normal'; going to work and parties and restaurants, over-eating crisps in parks with friends and attending 'character-building' hen parties with seventeen drunk strangers in foreign cities. I went to festivals and on holidays and made jokes and had fun with my friends and my wonderful family, and just exhaled into exhaustion and tears behind closed doors and tried to pretend everything was fine.

The thing is, you can try to ignore depression for your entire life, but at some point, the demons will have managed to sneak their way entirely into you and you won't be able to just close the door on them anymore. It's still up for debate as to whether depression can ever truly leave you, but the cold, hard fact is that it sticks around for a long time.

Depression's often talked about as 'just like any other illness, you wouldn't tell someone to get over pneumonia or a broken leg, would you! LOLs!' but in reality, of course, it's nothing like pneumonia or a broken leg, and I'd bet that most people with depression would give up an actual leg entirely if it meant that depression would bugger off forever.

When I got to the stage of being unable to ignore what was happening to me, it was because of the physical symptoms that had manifested, far more than it was because of the mental. Which is odd, because no one really talks about them. Depression is so much more than a mental struggle, and I didn't realize that all these bizarre things that were happening to my body were a result of an illness that had decided to plant itself in my brain. I was surprised to get a depression diagnosis; I thought I was just a bit sad.

Depression is a knackering little trollop, to put it lightly, and the fact that it disguises itself as part of your personality makes it all the more difficult to address. But address it we must – and we don't need to be polite about it. Nowadays, depression is very much still a part of my life, but in a much more manageable place. Accepting that it's sitting alongside me rather than just ignoring it and hoping it will just go away has made all the difference. By acknowledging it and trying to become more self-aware, I've figured out ways to live with it, and there really are times when I feel like it's not a part of me at all. When I was at my lowest, I could barely believe the 'vibrant' or even 'out of bed' person I used to be was real, never mind entertaining the thought that I would ever feel 'normal' again. But there is no normal. Mood, mindset and feelings are all on a sliding scale and 'within a normal range' does not exist.

I now feel like I have way more of a grip on it, and can separate the illness from myself and prepare to manage it more than I previously could. This book is what I needed to read when I first started feeling depressed and I sincerely hope it helps you or someone you love to try to understand this illness. In reading it, I hope to make those with depression in their lives feel more 'YES, OMG, ME TOO' and less 'Oh, nobody understands my misery and I'm a sad freak.'

When I first read a book about depression I felt like I wanted to rip out the pages and eat them because I related to some of the passages so much, in a way I'd never felt understood before. It was assuring and relieving and overwhelming to see my experiences almost exactly recreated on a page, and to feel like I wasn't the only one going mad. Of course, not every passage struck a chord as everyone's mental health is different, and I hope that this book will strike different chords with you as a sufferer, a carer, or someone just trying to understand the complexity of mental health struggles a bit more. You can of course eat the pages if you'd like.

I know that people I love will read this and might be shocked, and people who might be trying to learn about depression may also read this and be shocked – but I'm deeply afraid it will be for the wrong reasons. I want to clarify that I talk about wanting to die, a lot. As you'll learn as you read, or maybe understand if you've felt it too, this 'wanting to die' does not stem from hating everybody in my life and never wanting to see them again. It's not from finding my friends and family so intolerable that I want to leave them forever. It's about feeling such bulging sadness that I just want it to stop. Wanting to die is not the same as actively planning to end your life. I don't feel like this anymore due to the help of many things I mention in this book, and really want to stress that no person is to blame. It's just some weird head shit.

There are 'jokes' in this, and I try to laugh at depression a lot. It's great to be able to laugh (especially at your bullies), and if you're soaking up depression like a sad ol' sponge then I'm sure you've had periods of your life when you were *unable* to laugh. Depression is absolutely ridiculous in its absurdity and the way it messes you up in such contradictory ways. So why not take the low road and make fun of it? What are we without laughter, hey? Dullards. Lord knows we're definitely all dullards if we're depressed, so let's meet our demons and point at them and laugh.

Then you can go back to crying, that's absolutely OK.

CHAPTER 1

Just try some positive thinking, sweetie

'Come on, go out with me tonight. Staying home and thinking about your depression isn't going to help you, is it?'

There is an astonishing amount of people who seem to think that depression is just the result of us wallowing in our negative thoughts and indulging ourselves in self-hatred. If only this was better publicized and we knew that *not thinking about depression* would fix it. Let me think of flowers and butterscotch and daisies and doilies for a minute and I'll be right with you when I'm cured.

Everyone's got a new practice to wang on about these days, whether it's mindfulness or meditation, affirmations or astrology (birth charts do not help with mental health so you can just fuck right off with that suggestion, Susan). There's a whole bunch of noise about how to feel quiet, and of course everyone is wired differently and thus will find different methods of success. The suggestions can seem overwhelming, and the success rates are so varied. Being as over-connected as we love to be, we can now meditate using our phones, practise mindfulness on Instagram and scroll through endless WebMD articles about how to retrain our brains to think more positively. It's exhausting.

Meditation is constantly held up as the Oscar winner of the mindfulness game, but personally, I've never been able to do it in its traditional sense. Connecting to my thoughts for three minutes a morning will not cure anything for me, as my thoughts are a pile of toxic waste at the end of a dark tunnel. Surrounded by demons. On fire.

Sitting still and trying to quieten the mind will put me into a deeper depressive state than I was before, as there's nothing going on to distract me from the gloom.

Being told to think more positively suggests that you're *choosing* to be depressed, and that all depression really is a collection of your bad thoughts that you're actively dwelling on rather than quite easily living a cheery life by simply not allowing these thoughts to enter your head.

I didn't speak to anybody about sadness or negative thoughts before I was diagnosed with depression, and even then, it took a few months before I felt comfortable to bring it up with my family, and a few more years for everyone else. The 'cheer up' comments now come from 'friends' and are along the lines of 'Well, you're not going to feel any better if you stay in and think about it all night, are you?' in response to me cancelling plans because I feel too low, tired or sick.

I didn't realize depression could make you feel sick, but it turns out this is very much the case when it comes to mess you up with its pal, anxiety. In the UK you're actually four times more likely to have anxiety and depression together,[4] rather than having one alone, and anxiety can also occur as one of the symptoms of major clinical depression.[5] Cool.

Experts reckon anxiety and depression could be variations of the same disorder,[6] influenced by the happenings in our amygdala, which is the emotional centre of the brain and affects all its other parts.

A few years ago I unknowingly experienced the absolute riot of depression and anxiety at the same time, which truly made me feel like I was going completely mad and would have to be 'taken away and locked up' if I told anyone about it. Also, you can experience Mixed Anxiety-Depressive Disorder, which is bound to be just as fun as it sounds.

My particular bout of anxiety manifested in an overwhelming fear of everybody I love dying at any moment – and when I say overwhelming, I mean it was physically overwhelming to the stage that I had many invasive tests in many hospitals to try to work out what was wrong with my body. Turns out, anxiety and depression combo! Would you like fries with that?

I was sad all the time, and feeling hopeless, but I didn't seek any help for those feelings as I thought they were 'just my feelings' and that I should get a grip and get over them. The physical symptoms felt far more out of my control, though, so I did seek medical help for those.

I first noticed something happening physically when I started experiencing extreme bouts of dizziness and light-headedness. It would often feel like my surroundings were swimming around me, and that my head was full of helium and I could fall over at any moment. I found myself steadying myself for balance while sitting down at my desk. I would have to hold onto railings and bannisters everywhere I went for fear of absolutely stacking it, and generally spent life feeling as if I was on a boat.

I took a lot of medication to try to squash this dizziness, and remember realizing it wasn't working when I was sitting down in a café (in Italy, check me out) and gripping the table so tightly that while my knuckles turned white I was convinced I was about to fall backwards in my chair and take the table with me, and I was completely and utterly powerless to stop it.

So I went to the doctors, they did some examining and then sent me to the hospital for an MRI scan of my brain. If you've not had an MRI scan before, it's like being in a very loud, shuddering coffin that's vibrating with force as it scans your insides to find the tumours; 3/10, would not go again.

As I lay in the magnetic tube wondering if I actually did have some kind of metal in my guts that I'd forgotten about and that was about to be ripped out of my insides by the machine, I remember thinking, 'Fine, this is it, I have a brain tumour and will be dead soon.' (Depression and anxiety are very dramatic and self-indulgent, aren't they?) I thought, 'Brain cancer kills people quite quickly, right?' Certainly if *Grey's Anatomy* is anything to go by (and it IS) then I should be out of here in no time if I refuse treatment, and might get to have hot imaginary sex with a dead person's ghost in the meantime (you really have to have watched the show to understand that one, I don't have the inclination to explain it to you here). Brain cancer would be a good outcome, because then I would die and it *wouldn't be my fault* and nobody would be able to say that I was selfish to die or that I had done it because I didn't care about them. Brain cancer would be perfect.

But I didn't have brain cancer. I didn't have anything out of the ordinary that showed up on the MRI scan, and when the kind doctor told me that everything was completely normal with my brain, I didn't realize I was silently crying a steady flood of tears until she put her hand on my arm and said, 'But, darling, this is good news. What's wrong?'

It was this thoughtful doctor who first suggested to me that I might be depressed and anxious. She didn't say it to my face, because I was just sitting in front of her like a blubbering, quivering, weird pink mess (you know how your face gets all hot and blotchy when you cry?). She wrote it in my notes, which I received through the post about a week later.

'Kate's scan showed her brain to be healthy,' the note said, 'but I would encourage you to treat her for depression and anxiety, which I think may be the root cause. She certainly seemed quite teary when she was with me.'

'Quite teary.'

I put the notes away in a drawer, ashamed of wasting a doctor's time because I couldn't just get a grip on myself (as I kept telling myself to do), as I physically tried to get myself a grip on the kitchen counter because I thought I was about to fall over again.

Before the dizziness came along, I was in hospital another time for an intimate examination of my stomach and digestive system after I'd returned to London from four months of travelling and doctors thought I might have caught some kind of tropical disease.

It started because I thought I was pregnant, having felt cripplingly nauseous every morning to the point of actual vomiting about 50 per cent of the time. I don't even know if I was having sex at this point, but being pregnant is the only explanation for morning sickness, right? But the sickness lasted all day, and it chewed up my stomach and rose up into my throat and also gave me really weird poo, to be honest.

I saw the doctor (as I looked at my online booking confirmation I did not realize that this was my seventh appointment in four weeks), who referred me to hospital for an upper endoscopy. This is an examination where a tube with a teeny camera on the end of it is pushed down your throat and into your stomach so that the doctors can examine your digestive tract and the upper part of your small intestine. Not wanting to drag anyone else into it, I opted for the 'being wide awake' version of the examination, as having sedation meant many more hours in recovery and having to be accompanied by someone else when the time came to leave the hospital.

I don't know if you've ever had a tube put down your throat, but 'not very pleasant' isn't exactly the phrase I would choose to describe it. 'Abso-fucking-lutely fucking horrific' is closer to the mark, as you lie on your left side in a hospital theatre while a Medical Marvel (I don't know if they were a nurse or a doctor or what, and don't want to get it wrong, and it's fair to assume that everyone who works for the NHS is a Medical Marvel and shall just be referred to as MM in future times of my confusion, many thanks) is holding you down firmly with one hand pressed flat on your hip and the other on your shoulder, because you're about to quite violently retch.

Another MM puts a plastic mouth guard around the inside of your lips, keeping your mouth pushed open a bit like the world's most unappealing sex doll. Another MM (I didn't realize until it was nearly over), just stays with you and holds your hand.

A moment for the hand-holding, please.

The tube – which I remember being the girth and length of a full-grown python but was probably really more like a garden hose – is then pushed into your mouth and down your throat, and the heaving and retching begins. Astonishingly there was no vomit, just a loooottt of saliva, but that feeling of the tube being pushed further down as your body tries to more forcefully reject it was a series of hot, scratchy convulsions that really didn't stand up to the 'pre-examination numbing throat spray'.

(Side note, I had a friend who had a lower endoscopy – where the camera goes up your arse – and who perhaps quite wisely opted to accept the sedation before the procedure. She described it as 'like having two or three large glasses of white wine, and after that you don't really care about what goes up yer arse, do you?')

Anyway, once the end of the tube has got past the tricky bit in your throat, you just need to remember to breathe (an MM will remind you) and enjoy the heaving, retches and alarmingly loud guttural burps that come with every teeny movement of the camera inside you. Same thing all over again when it comes back up, and the poor, sweet MM who's holding your hand has likely lost all feeling in *their* hand with your sweaty, shaky, crushing hold. It's short, about fifteen minutes, and fifteen minutes of feeling intensely like you're just about to spew would be nothing if it could lead to the reason why I felt like I was about to spew every day. If the MMs could just find what was in there that was messing up my guts.

They found nothing. Of course they found nothing.

There's a reason that the phrase 'gut feeling' exists; our brains are connected to everything – of course, they're the master controller extraordinaire of everything about us, but it turns out our brains and our gastrointestinal systems are actually directly linked. This is why when you're stressed, your body releases more of the 'stress hormone', cortisol, in your stomach, and why people can then get stress-induced stomach ulcers

SAME FOR DEPRESSION. How fun! Depression can affect the movements of your GI tract,[7] which means hello, feelings of extreme sickness and days of totally wild poop. A Norwegian study found that depression and anxiety were significantly higher in people experiencing heavy nausea,[8] and my experience shows it to certainly have been true for me.

Dizziness, as I discovered after the trip to the MRI-doom-tube and various appointments with ear doctors to check if my hearing and balance were to blame for me walking into everything (one week I fell over on the way to work EVERY DAY, and I hadn't even been spiking my morning coffee with Baileys) and clumsiness are also physical symptoms of depression and anxiety. Not much has been 'officially' investigated about the link, but there are studies that suggest that some people with vertigo or dizziness may have it as a result of depression.[9]

Here are some more fun physical elements of depression that I and others have experienced:

- **Shaky hands**. Like those of a very aged person, in an old British sitcom, trying to carry a tray of tea to a group.
- **Heavy, aching muscles**. Muscles that hurt as though you've been in Beast Mode at the gym, when the reality is more like the total opposite.
- **Extreme lethargy and a constant need for sleep**. Spending long days in bed thinking, 'One more nap and I'll be able to get up'… infinitely.
- **Extreme sensitivity to noise**. Loud noises can make me cry.
- **Absolutely no libido whatsoever**. None. Squat. Nada. No sex for me, please. Horrible stuff. I'm not a pervert.
- **Increased sexual arousal**. Depression is nice and contradictory, so whereas it can affect your libido by taking it away, it can also heighten your sexual 'interest', shall we say. When

the brain discovers that the sexy bit is way more interesting than the sad bit, and that when the sexy bit lights up it's so bright and noisy that it can even make the sad bit be quiet for a while.

- **Slo-mo movements.** This one is weird, especially for a person who loves to walk fast and is constantly in direct competition with Google Maps, which thinks it'll take you seventeen minutes to walk somewhere but you *know* you can do it in twelve. Suddenly it's like your body has given up the first-place position to the Googz, as you walk like you're wading through waist-deep mud at Glastonbury but without all the face-glitter.

- **Chest pain.** I think this one blesses those with either depression or anxiety, and for me it felt like a sharp twang right in the middle of my breastbone that once made me tell my then-boyfriend, 'If I collapse in this restaurant, I was having chest pains so it's probably a heart attack – just so you know.' A friend told me that his chest pains feel like someone's put a rope around his chest and is trying to pull it forcefully to his back. Another friend (yeah, I move in some pretty sad circles) said that their chest pain takes the form of thumping heart palpitations that they're convinced everyone can hear. We can't.

Another LOLsome thing about being a Girl (Interrupted) is that you have a whole other whack of 'interesting' reproductive plumbing that can also decide to pack it in if you're depressed. Bodies are amazing, really, and will stop producing eggs if they're in distress because, hey, you probably shouldn't have a kid if you can't cope with life (when will we all realize that the world is on fire and just give up with the reproductive lark altogether? Eh?).

My plumbing decided to quit the egg scene when I was feeling abominably dark. Not that I was in the mood for shagging anyway, but my body decided outright that I was such a mess it would be an unspeakable disaster to reproduce me in any way. Well done, body. Obviously, despite the lack of sex your first thought when you miss a period is 'OMG fuckssaaaaakehowcanIbepregnantomg it's happening', but after many tests to confirm that, yet again, I was not with child, I headed back off to the ol' doc's office after three bloodless months.

Does anyone's doctor do loyalty cards?

So, more tests, which involved blood samples and one of those very-fucking-cold ultrasounds that they do from inside your vagina, which is a bit like how I imagine it would feel to have someone shoving a magic ultrasound dildo up you and making concerned noises while swabbing it around like a thirteen-year-old boy playing with a light sabre having his first go at foreplay.

Of course, they found nothing, but a few blood tests later showed that I had a monstrously elevated level of prolactin; a hormone created by the pituitary gland in your brain. I was shown on the leaflet handed to me by the doc that if an excessive amount of prolactin is squirted out (OK probably not squirted, as such) then it's likely because you have a prolactinoma – which is just as fun as it sounds. A prolactinoma is a non-cancerous tumour in your brain right on that particular gland that causes accidental pressure on the 'press here for prolactin' button.

I had NEVER heard of this hormone before, and upon further research it seems that it's pretty famous among the breastfeeding crowds because of its link to milk production, but that it's also linked to depression. People don't really know how yet, because money never goes towards research into female medical conditions when it could go towards *viagra* and erectile dysfunction. I digress.

It's a bit of a chicken-and-egg situation with prolactin and depression (there's an egg joke in there somewhere... but I can't quite reach it. Answers on a postcard, please) and 'they' don't yet know if the depression comes first and causes the prolactin party, or if the prolactin party starts and depression is the first name on the guest list.

The elaborate point I'm trying to make here is that depression is NOT just about positive or negative thinking. It's more than something 'all in your head' and can in fact show itself as a deep-fried buffet of physical strangeness served all over your body before you even begin to realize that your brain isn't working as it should be.

Depression is not just about your thoughts.

Depression is a medical illness that manifests in physical and mental symptoms. It's the mental symptoms that end up giving it such a complex and stigmatized reputation, and that end up leading people to think that they can make you better if they just love you harder. It's heartbreaking to see people you love blame themselves for your illness, or try to fix it for you when you know that it's so, so much bigger than they are. We're not all Harry Potter, we can't all be protected by love.

Rather than practising meditation or some other spiritual flapdoodle that will leave me alone with my own thoughts, I find that absorbing myself completely in something else can hush up the brain demons for a bit – but of course this will vary depending on how hard the demons are working at that point.

In fact, some studies have shown that distraction is a valid way of lessening depressive thoughts. Putting your energy into focusing on something else that isn't your pain will construct your brain stimulus so that pain is no longer at the forefront of your attentional systems. When you're in a rich and stimulating environment, pain signals in the brain are diminished. Those with less going on around them are more likely to feel mental pain.[10]

Not being able to read properly was one of the most distressing periods I had, because if I couldn't hide from the world in a book then where else could I go? Reading and re-reading sentences over and over again doesn't lend itself to total absorption, so at that point I really did feel like I was fucked. I don't know if you've ever tried to read while in an all-consuming depressive state – I assume you have, seeing as you picked up this book (tick) about depression (tick). Don't you find the words kind of fuzz up as you look at them? If you finally get to the end of a few lines, you've forgotten what the first ones said anyway, so then you have to go back over and over. Then the ink darkens and the page softens and you didn't even realize you were crying onto it. It's horrible.

If your brain is being left alone enough to the point that you can actively consume outside words and the thoughts of others (yay!) then I'd implore you to read a book, listen to a podcast, or even stoop to my levels of elderly comforts and find yourself a window-box to tend and do some gardening.

Keeping a full and busy mind certainly works for me when I can find the motivation to do it. Stuffing it with compelling television, articles, books or music is far more preferable than trying to be still and silent, for me. Neuroscientist Dr Daniel Levitin conducted a study that showed that listening to music activates the same reward centres in the brain that are activated when we have meaningful social interactions, which suggests that music really can save lives and help stem feelings of loneliness or misery.

But is busying your mind with stories from books and films and twenty-five hours of a TV show actually healthy? At this point I'm not entirely sure I give a damn. If there's something that can temporarily release the demons back into the wild world outside of my brain and distract me with a gripping tale of horrific true crime instead, marvellous.

Mindfulness is about 'being present'. That sounds so trite and American, but sometimes there just aren't better words that sum something up.

In fact, I've recently learned that mindfulness isn't about skipping through meadows of corn, hugging trees and doing 'ommmmm' chants. Instead, Kate Mason describes it as 'about being in the moment and noticing your thoughts and physical feelings and surroundings. Kids are amazing at doing this, it's only through societal pressures and demands as we move into adulthood that we lose the ability to be in the moment – we're always looking ahead, which can instil anxiety, or looking into the past, which can instil depression.'

Aren't grown-ups fun?

The good thing about mindfulness is it's not something that you either can or cannot do, like licking your elbow. Mindfulness can be learned and practised and finessed. Kate is a big advocate of 'the 5-4-3-2-1 technique', which can help you to practise being present and 'in the moment'. If you'd like to have a crack, it goes as follows:

Name five things you can see at this very moment, four things you can hear, three things you can feel (like your feet in your shoes or your bum on a chair), two things you can smell and one thing you can taste, even if it's just the inside of your mouth or a sip of cold water.

I use this technique sometimes when I'm feeling overwhelmed with pretty much any emotion: sadness, anger, stress – you name it. Sometimes I forget the number part though (sorry, Kate) and just try to focus on what I can see, feel and smell, and to have some water. It certainly helps calm me down and bring me more into focus.

So, you can't think your way out of depression, but you can start to try and train yourself to be able to manage the depression you have. Accepting that you aren't entirely well and that you can't carry on pretending everything is fine is really the first step. Paying attention to what helps soothe or distract you is crucial, as is looking out for signs that you might be heading towards a depressive episode. If you can be aware of both of these things, you can try to combine the two superpowers to achieve the seemingly impossible: survive. Realizing that you can't make plans for every evening, or even just paying attention to what you have coming up in your schedule or life that might make you feel worse, so that you can then block out some time to decompress, helps. Get on your phone calendar and start colour-coding, emoji-ing or whatever it is you need to do to take some control.

The clapbacks

When someone fancies themselves as your Healer-in-Chief and makes a blithe suggestion about how you could better manage your mental health, it can be tricky to know how to respond. Sometimes, it really does come from a place of kindness and the person in question just doesn't have a clue how to help you. Other times, though, it can come from a place of smugness and in that case the person in question can... well... they can fuck off. I'll finish every chapter with a selection of clapbacks that you could say the next time some unsolicited advice is thrown at you.

Having somebody tell you to 'just try some positive thinking' is infuriating, so I encourage everyone to be as bitter and pedantic and problematic as possible because it just PISSES ME OFF SO MUCH.

'OK, OK, OK, hold my hands and do it with me... Sunshine, lollipops, rainbows... and friends who know that depression isn't just about how you think! Amazing. Thanks!'

'Wait, you mean that's all it takes? I just need to think back to when Britney and Justin were together and everything will be OK?'

'This is me being positive.' (More powerful when accompanied with very limp jazz hands.)

'Oh! I thought negative thinking would help me. Thank God you're here.'

If you're more mature than I am and would like to respond productively, I would suggest:

'Actually, depression affects me physically as well as mentally so it's not just about thoughts. I'm trying to use the lighter moments to get ready for the darker ones, though, which I can't control.'

CHAPTER 2

Just get some pills then, dear

Medication is often the first suggestion someone will bring to the table when told about a mental health problem, and it makes sense. Medication can cure a lot of other health problems, and if someone had tonsillitis you'd probably suggest antibiotics.

Of course, though, it's different for mental illnesses.

If you're considering opting for medication to help you with your depression, it's crucial to know that there are multiple options available – as well as drug-free options, talking therapies, cognitive behavioural therapy (CBT) and much more.

When I eventually went to the doctor after realizing I could be depressed, following the aforementioned hospital tests and many late nights spent hoping Google could solve my problems, medication was the first suggestion for me, alongside therapy.

I took the medication hungrily as I was so desperate for anything to make my brain feel better. I had to go through a few periods of trialling different kinds before I found the medicine that was the exact right one for me. Like Goldilocks! Of doom.

There is still a lot of stigma attached to taking medication for mental illness, as medication is seen to just treat the surface of the problem and not solve 'the real issues' behind mental health problems. When a friend went to therapy for his severe anger problems and was prescribed medication, I was quick to slag off the doctor for avoiding 'the real issue' and for turning so quickly to pharma. Did the psychiatrist not want to talk about his issues, I wondered? Did the psychiatrist just want to do the easy thing and throw dangerous medication at him, which could bring out all kinds of side effects? I was projecting the very same stigma that I try to abolish – even those of us who know the benefits and advantages of medication have been conditioned into automatically thinking it's the devil.

But taking medication for my depression has made me more able to deal with and prepare for depressive episodes, so who's to say the anger medication won't do the same for the red mist. You can see it from both sides, really.

There's nothing bad about taking medication for depression. Even that sentence sounds so obvious you wouldn't think I had to write it down. The bit that I'm conflicted about is the stage at which meds are introduced to people, and how they are explained and monitored. I know medication works. If it works for you, keep taking it! I have no plans to come off my medicine and have been taking it for years.

Without the medication I can't get out of bed. Without the medication I can't physically or mentally focus on anything apart from the darkness. The only thought rolling around my mind is that this all has to end and how can I make it end and why hasn't it ended yet (um, because you're just lying in bed in the dark and not doing anything about it, love)? Without the medication, the dizziness and the nausea came back, along with the excruciating headaches and seemingly a complete intolerance to alcohol. I was basically a wobbling, vomiting, head-holding drunk.

The medication didn't fix my depression at all, but it cleared the road of a whole load of shit I didn't even realize was in the way before I started taking medication. I was still depressed, but I was less consumed by it. To continue the weather metaphors, I and others have described the effects of antidepressants as like a fog being lifted; it's still grey and rainy, but you can actually see the roads ahead of you now rather than having no sight of what's ahead.

But antidepressants are a bit like the contraceptive pill (or, if you're a biological male reading this, perhaps I could liken them to getting a Starbucks order exactly right after countless adjustments and changes to see what your perfect concoction is). There are *so many* types of antidepressants available, they all take a fair whack of time to properly kick in (at least three weeks), and they all have different effects on different people depending on what mixture of brain and body chemistry they're faced with post-swallow (steady on).

After I'd gone through the tests in the hospital, found nothing and continued to be miserable, I finally conceded to the idea that maybe I might be depressed. Of course, this manifested in the modern way of lying awake in the wee hours of the morning, googling 'how to know if you're depressed' on my phone and taking an NHS quiz to try to self-diagnose.

Even the quiz was traumatizing, and I found myself in gushes and convulsions of tears as I selected a frequency for how often I experienced things such as 'feeling bad about yourself, or that you are a failure, or have let yourself or your family down?' and realizing that it was constantly. All the time. All day, every sodding day. It's quite startling to see it laid out in front of you like that.

After reaching the results screen that essentially said WOAH, HEY, ARE YOU THE GRIM REAPER? I thought I should probably go to the doctor about it.

My appointment came around the next week. When I got to the doctor's surgery, I sat in the waiting room feeling waves of shame that didn't stop crashing. What was I doing, taking up an appointment slot when there were people who actually had real illnesses and needed urgent care? What was I going to say, 'I can't stop feeling sad'? Why waste the NHS's valuable and already stretched time with that? Just cheer up.

Surely I'm not actually depressed enough, anyway, and the doctor will tell me to pull myself together and get a grip. Will they think I'm pretending just to get some drugs? *Am I pretending? Is this even real?*

I was about to leave and stood up just as my name beeped onto the screen. I figured it would be an even bigger waste of their time to actually not go into the appointment I'd booked, so I traipsed to Room 3 and did that performative knock you do even though you know the doctor is expecting you, and you're not exactly 'just in the area and thought you would pop by'.

I walked in and sat down, and the doctor asked me why I was here. 'I... um...' Breathe. 'I think I'm depressed,' I said, for the first time ever, out loud. And then the crying came, and it wouldn't stop. It was the crying that a child does when it's fallen over, the kind that makes you sound like a baboon when you try to inhale because you kind of choke on your own breath.

The doctor passed me a box of tissues and I tried, limply, to soak up rivers of tears and snot.

'Why do you think that?' he asked, softly.

I couldn't speak. I couldn't do anything except cry. It was so shameful, and childlike, and useless, and probably disrespectful to his medical degree, but I just sat in his chair and half hyperventilated and half sobbed. I managed to get out an 'I… [sob]… feel… [choke]… like… [sob]… this… [sob]… everysingledayallthetime.' He wrote me a prescription for sertraline and I shuffled out of the room, feeling about four years old. Didn't even get a bloody sticker.

I took the sertraline, and at first noticed no difference apart from maybe the possibility that I was potentially getting wobblier on my feet. A few weeks into the treatment, my boyfriend noticed that I was leaning a hand on every available surface in the flat as I made my way from the sofa to the bathroom (such is the life of an athlete) and was looking to balance myself wherever I could. 'I'm just tired,' I told him. 'It feels like I could fall asleep at any moment.' I washed my face in the bathroom, noting in the mirror that my eyes were dilated to an almost cartoonish level of wideness. My pupils looked like 2p coins.

The doctor had only prescribed a month of treatment, so I had to make an appointment to go back and review how it had been. Now, here's where I know I'm lucky that I was a) able to make an appointment for around the time I needed one, and didn't have to wait for weeks, and b) in the headspace where I actually made an appointment. If I hadn't gone back, and had let the tiny amount of sertraline in my system wear off, and continued to be depressed and maybe even killed myself, would anyone in that doctor's surgery know? Do they have to know? Are they meant to be aware of their patients' trajectories like this or am I putting too much pressure on them? We all know that NHS staff are stretched to their absolute limits, and I'm not blaming the individuals, I'm blaming… well, I guess I'm blaming the system, in particular, the admin.

It's easy to drop off, or slip through, or whatever you want to call it. If medication doesn't work for you and you can't bring yourself to go back, that'll be it. I had one friend who couldn't get an appointment to request more antidepressants so he weaned himself off them just two months after starting them. Yes, stop screaming at the page, I know you are able to request a repeat prescription online but a) he didn't know about this b) I'm not actually sure if you can do this after your very first trial on a medicine and c) it would have really helped to speak to someone about the side effects and effectiveness of the medication.

People can drop off so easily. Nobody called him to see how he was doing and I GET IT, there's nobody *to* call him.

So I went back to the doctor, tail between my legs, and told him that actually I still cry every day and don't see the point in living. I tried antidepressants and they made me unbalanced and didn't change anything else at ALL, so I guess I'm doomed now. Where do I get fitted for a straitjacket?

Oh no, no, no. There is not only one kind of antidepressant. This, at twenty-six, shouldn't have been shocking to me at all – but then again it was only yesterday (now that I am thirty-two) that I realized that Ross, Chandler and Joey from *Friends* all love *Die Hard*, and yet said nothing when Rachel starts going out with Bruce Willis. Twenty years ago. So it's fair to say that sometimes I'm slow on the uptake.

So this time I left with a prescription for citalopram and a pending appointment for a cognitive behavioural therapy session that would be sometime in the next four months, hopefully.

Citalopram. Wow. Citalopram knocked me the fuck OUT. Citalopram made me so tired I felt like I was made of wrought iron. I lost weight because I couldn't bring myself to move to eat anything. I lost days because I would stay in bed. I lost my sex drive completely, and at one point I swear I actually went completely numb between the legs and lost all the feeling in my vagina.

Well, that was it. If anything's gonna make you sadder than you already are, it's not being able to feel your vag. I stopped taking the citalopram and slowly got my energy back. This seemed to come at around the same time as my CBT appointment reared its questioning head, and – now this is just personal experience from how I felt and what I did and how it all made me feel, you get it, but what an absolute crock of shit.

I can see, really really see, that CBT would be tremendously useful if you have anxiety, anger issues, crippling self-doubt or something that presents itself in some kind of behavioural pattern. This is not how I experience my depression though, and CBT felt incredibly redundant when it was put against my demons.

'Tell me how you feel when you feel depressed', the chirpy therapist said, 'and write it in this bubble.'

'Like I want to die,' I wrote, and looked at her.

'Right! OK! Well, now in the next bubble, tell me what usually happens to make you feel like this.'

…I've got nothing. 'This is how I always feel,' I told her. 'Nothing happens to bring it on, it's just how I always feel.'

'OK!'

We tried a different approach.

'Tell me something that you're worried about,' she went on,

pulling out a fresh sheet of paper with a flourish. 'What's your biggest worry right now?'

'That I'm not going to be able to die soon and will spend my whole life feeling like this.'

'Right! OK! So, put that in the box that says "thoughts". Now, what would you say for the box that says "feelings"?'

… and so it went on. I reluctantly went back for one more session because I thought maybe there would be a different approach this time after the first appointment went so catastrophically sideways, but nope.

CBT is rigid; you assess your thoughts, your feelings, your physical reactions to things and your resulting behaviour that comes from you thinking these thoughts. Then you learn new behaviour patterns, and how to more effectively respond to potentially triggering situations. It helps you become acutely aware of your patterns of negative thought and gives you the mental tools to stop them. This can be so good for so many problems, but alas, I didn't find it helpful for my depression one teeny bit.

I was very much not at a stage where I felt comfortable talking about depression at all, and I found the direct approach of CBT quite intimidating. I had no idea where my depression was coming from and didn't have anything to put down in any twee little boxes. Talking about it made me feel ashamed, so it was a hard nope from me.

Also, I find that my depression doesn't really come with a negative thought 'process'. It's more like… just a constant, giant, negative energy that's crushing you further each time your heart dares to beat. When you're depressed, your 'reinforcement learning' doesn't quite work, and you reeeeally need that to be tip top if you're going to get anything from CBT.

I went back to the doctor. Eventually.

When sertraline and citalopram both turned out to be unhelpful (for me) and CBT made me feel stupid and guilty, I retreated back into my cave (by which I mean, my bed) in shame, feeling foolish for trying to draw any attention to anything in the first place.

I knew I should have another go when my mind started to affect my work. Not because I cared hugely about my job, but I did care somewhat about being able to pay rent, especially if I lost my job and then had no motivation to find another one.

I was taking a lot of 'work from home' days, which meant keeping my computer on and keeping Slack open while I cried in bed in the dark, or slept, or both. When I did make it out of bed to get to the office, I couldn't concentrate on anything. My eyes couldn't focus; numbers in spreadsheets all blurred together, and words on the screen meant nothing and had to be re-read countless times before I could actually absorb them. My mind was making me into an idiot.

So I went back to the doctor. He asked me if I had tried exercise, and I think I just stared at him with mild confusion on my face as a response. Exercise? Getting out of bed and leaving the house every day was like competing in an Ironman Triathlon (I assume). There was no way I could have ever found the energy to move around even more.

He wrote me a prescription for fluoxetine, starting on just 20mg. I trundled down to the nearby Boots and waited for my name to be called as I stared at a shelf of incontinence pads. I went back home and took a pill.

I took a pill every day for about three weeks, and nothing happened. I still felt as dark and as miserable as before but didn't have any annoying side effects. Was this just a placebo, I wondered?

Did I just pay £8 for a fake pill that does nothing because the doctor thought I was an attention-seeking liar, so just gave me something to make me go away?

I went back to the doctor (seriously, I think I must have had one of the most available surgeries in the UK) and told him, through tears, that the pills weren't helping. 'That's good news,' he said. Was he quite mad? 'If you've had no side effects, let's up the dose and see if that makes any difference.'

He has been to medical school, so I thought I'd just let that one slide.

Then a funny thing happened, but it crept up on me slowly so I couldn't see it happening, until one day, about a month later, I realized everything was different.

I was still depressed, don't get me wrong, but I wasn't spending the entire time in bed during work from home days – sometimes I even did a little work, because I could see properly again. My focus had come back and I was even *reading a book*. It was a book about depression because I was still utterly miserable, aching and hollow, but I could READ (it was Sally Brampton's *Shoot the Damn Dog*, if you're interested). It was while reading about not being able to read because of depression that I realized I was, in fact, reading those words. A feat that would have been unthinkable a few months ago and I was now doing it without even realizing.

Some of the fog had lifted without me noticing, and I think it was down to the medication. Well, I know it was.

I'm not trying to push a pro-drugs agenda on you, I'm just saying that after what seemed like a *lot* of time and effort, antidepressants helped me. I'm still on them today, although at a higher dose yet again – I think I've been taking them for about three or four years now. I tried to wean myself off them one summer when I thought I felt able to get by without them, and I absolutely could not. When they wore off, I was straight back to the darkness, literally and mentally, and the suicidal feelings were stronger than ever before. I went back on them.

Why do we think that we shouldn't need to rely on medicine? It is one of the miracles of the modern world that we have scientific advancements made purely to make us feel better. I really hate comparing depression or mental illnesses to any other purely physical illness, because honestly, they're so different it doesn't seem fair to either of them.

Medication helps me but has not cured me. A combination of medication, some exercise (I KNOW, eventually) and talking therapy has made me able to manage my mental health – but I wouldn't have had the headspace to bring exercise or therapy into my iPhone calendar if I didn't take the meds in the first place.

There is still a lot of stigma about antidepressants, just as there is about depression itself. A lot of people think that we're living in a world where people choose 'the easy way out' or the 'cheating route' of medication, without addressing any of the 'real issues'. Yes, my doctor seemed quick to write a prescription for pharmaceuticals, but it was the drugs that cleared the pathway to be able to think more clearly and take steps towards coping.

Psychiatry registrar Dr Ken Adams was kind enough to talk to me about prescribing antidepressants:

Antidepressants can of course have a placebo effect, and because physical health conditions are usually treated with medications, I think people are led to think that a similar model exists for treating depression, i.e. there is a pill to make it better. This means that there can be pressure on doctors to prescribe. Even as psychiatrists, we find it hard to tell patients that they do not need to be on medications – we find this a lot in the treatment of personality disorders when the evidence is in favour of psychological approaches, and the evidence base for medications is slim.

But how do you know if medication is something you should look into? I'd say that if you're even wondering about it, then it means you probably should. If you've been thinking about it to yourself, then why not think about it out loud to a doctor, and they can give you some clarity, answers and advice.

So here I am on my fluoxetine and not dead. Neither am I falling over all the time like I was with sertraline, or too tired and heavy to move at all like with citalopram – but it does come with its own side effects. I'm lucky, in that the only side effects it seems to have on me is an extreme thirst – drinking lots of water is hardly a bad thing – and it's made it harder to have an orgasm, but who doesn't like a vaginal challenge?

The list of potential side effects, though, almost put me off completely (I say almost because, despite their capacity to be severe, it felt worth the risk to be able to fix my head). To be fair, if you read the lists of potential side effects of any medication you'll probably want to just drink some bleach instead, but antidepressants seem to have their own particular list of potentials that are a) contradictory, b) seem to be the thing you're trying to use the medication to get rid of in the first place and c) fucking horrific.

One of the most fun, perhaps, is that antidepressants can cause an increase in suicidal thoughts if you have clinical depression. WHAT THE ACTUAL SHITTERY IS THIS? You could take medication for your misery, feel even more miserable and off yourself anyway? That doesn't really seem like a good use of anyone's time. Well done, everyone.

As well as increased depression, increased anxiety, potential lethargy, increased appetite, loss of appetite (covering all the bases there), purple spots on the skin, red eyes, rapid weight gain, blue–yellow colour blindness (?!what?!), decreased vision, severe sleepiness, a *large hive-like swelling on the face*, fainting, vomiting blood, unusual or incomplete body movements (again, what?!), the lists of potential side effects often include the following:

- **No blood pressure or pulse**
- **Stopping of the heart**

Which I'm sure you'll agree are 'quite severe'. But I was at the stage where I was willing to try anything to make the darkness lift, and the slim chance of developing a temporary new beehive-face didn't bother me. What's the point of having a face like a face if you spend your whole life miserable? Would rather take vomiting blood, fainting, weird body movements and my face turning into the Elephant Man if it meant that the depression would go away. The possibility of 'no blood pressure or pulse' without being dead would be quite fun at parties, and the potential heart-stopping… well, it seemed less likely to happen than the potential lessening of my depression, so I went for it.

When I experienced the side effects from the first two kinds of antidepressants I tried, I was still completely miserable, so I didn't see the point of having the side effects for no reason. If I felt the gloom ebbing away, though, I could definitely handle falling over all the time. Would just have to buy knee pads.

I asked the people of the internet for their 'inconvenient' anti-depressant side effects that under most other circumstances you would definitely quit your meds for, but that are actually better than having your depression be as bad as it was before you took the medication. Here's some of what they told me:

- 'Seriously sweaty palms. I need a desk fan to try and dry them when I'm at the office. They flare up all morning, every single day.'
- 'I get hot flushes *all* the time, and a constant, very dry mouth.'
- 'Honestly? It's really hard to get off. I have the same libido but just... a loss of sensation in my vagina. The mental health benefits far outweigh the 60 per cent reduction in orgasms, though.'
- 'More anxiety, which can make me so dizzy that I see white spots.'
- 'Hives! Actual hives on my arms, chest, neck and back, which is really awkward when I'm at work. I have to take antihistamines to counteract them, which in turn make me really drowsy.'
- 'My muscles twitch all day and it's exhausting as well as weird. My blood pressure is lower on the medicine, so I feel tired very easily and sometimes pass out.'

The good news (FINALLY) is that these medications aren't addictive. But if you come off them then you're pretty likely to experience withdrawal symptoms. When I foolishly thought that my depression seemed to be in check and that I probably didn't need medication anymore 'because I could handle it myself',

I stopped taking my fluoxetine for a period that I now refer to as The Summer of Doom. I weaned myself off them so, so gradually, but I still got the headaches, these brain-zap things and – oh yeah, the depression.

Man, was I relieved to google 'brain electrocuted body fizzing what why?' and find that brain zaps are indeed 'a thing'; they're also sometimes called brain shivers or brain flips. Basically, you can be walking to the kettle like you always do, and then BZZZZAAAAPPP, your brain has had a police taser zapped onto it. It's alarming, and so different from a headache in that you really only feel it on your actual brain, not your skull or muscle or tissue or whatever it is between your brain and the outside of your face. Just your brain.

The BZZZZZAAAAPPP on my brain then shot down each arm like a lightning rod and ended up fizzing into my hands like pins and needles, if pins and/or needles were dancing like a Cossack in my veins.

There hasn't been a whole load of research into what causes the zaps, although there are some medics who say that the zaps are linked to 'lateral eye movements', i.e. when we look anywhere but straight ahead. Brilliant. If you're planning to wean yourself off your antidepressants, do ensure you invest in a good pair of blinkers.

When I was coming off the medication, I was also the crankiest gal in town. The Ultimate Queen of Strops. I was Ursula the sea witch but watching *The Apprentice*. On her period. Surrounded by screaming children. Can octopus-people get periods? Not the point. I was way beyond 'irritable', I was annoyed at everything and everyone, and it turns out that the annoyance highway was actually right en route back to depressionville.

This was me weaning myself off at an infuriatingly slow rate. Stopping the medication cold-turkey would have been horrific. PLEASE DON'T DO IT. The weird stigma that we have about taking antidepressants is another completely unnecessary modern load of shite. If they help you, they help you. If you think you're cured, that may well be because of the medication. If you want to see how true that is then for the love of Rihanna please go see your doctor and take their advice. Come off them so, so slowly, and be ready for a potential collapse. You'll need to make sure you tell people who spend a lot of time with you that you're making some changes in medication (you don't have to be specific if you'd rather not hit them with a 'Surprise! I'm depressed! I think! Maybe not anymore! Let's all watch ahahaha!') so they can look out for you and help pull you out of the quicksand if you find yourself back in there.

If you're keen to explore obtaining drugs from your health provider that can help manage your mental health illness, here are a few things to remember:

- There are many types of antidepressant medication available. Ask your doctor to talk through what the options are, and what they could be if your first 'go' doesn't give you the desired effects.
- These pills take time. It's not like having a paracetamol for a headache, it's like the prank where you move your boss's desk by an inch every day until one day they realize they're in a totally different place.
- Medication will not fix you, but it may alleviate some of the pain. It will not make your days sunny, but it will clear

a lot of the fog. You won't be healed because you've had medicine, but you'll eventually start to see the shape of the path you need to take to get there. You won't (or are very unlikely to, anyway) feel completely 'cured' – use the lighter moments to try to prepare for when the darker moments come back.

The clapbacks

When someone suggests that you try antidepressants and you have absolutely no idea what to say back, perhaps try one of these:

'I'd like to try other approaches first, but I know that they're an option.'

'It's something I'm thinking about, but I know they won't fix everything.'

'I do. I am. This is me with my head above the water.'

'Shame they don't make pills for unsolicited advice, isn't it?'

CHAPTER 3

Can't you take 'shrooms
for that now, pet?

As we live in the age of the internet and everyone seems to enjoy trying stuff and then writing about it online, we now have access to hundreds of personal experiences, studies and papers about other, non-pharmaceutical medication options for depression. By which I mean drrruggy drug drugs.

One of my favourite schools of thought, and perhaps the most promising (but alas, least tasty), is that a chemical compound called psilocybin can provide effective relief from depression. The research and studies have moved on so much in the last few years that there are now those who reckon that psilocybin doesn't just treat depression, but could actually *cure* depression. A depression cure. Gulp.

Psilocybin is the psychoactive ingredient that puts the magic in magic mushrooms, and my curiosity around it and 'alternative treatments' was roused after I took them and felt *truly* magical. That day, I'd had no idea how many mushrooms were too many mushrooms, so I decided to be Captain Sensible and slowly graze on them.

It was the happiest I've felt in years.

Everything felt lighter. If my regular functioning levels had always been at -25, now I'd finally reached the baseline of 0. The depression gremlins had been replaced with a bit of sparkle. Since then, my excitement has taken me into the depths of scientific studies, and led to me taking up the time of some very generous experts who further enlightened me on the benefits of psilocybin for our mental health. I landed upon some fascinating information about psilocybin *and* some other drugs you absolutely would not get from your doctor, and obviously I wanted to share my findings with you in case they might be helpful.

The (p)science behind psilocybin

The Synthesis Institute (a respected company based in the Netherlands) describes the effects of psilocybin very well (as they should, being a leading researcher into the stuff) and says that 'by altering several different neurotransmitter systems in the brain, magic mushrooms or truffles activate serotonergic receptors on neurons, causing several brain systems to significantly change, and a wave of unique excitatory activity to spread throughout the main perceptual centres of the mind.'

In less scientific talk, this essentially means that shrooms make you feel elated joy and happiness. Depending on the dosage, they can change your vision, make you super introspective, or just make you feel like you're floating around on a sparkly skateboard, throwing love to everyone you pass by, like a little flower girl of delight.

Studies have shown that psilocybin has provided relief from and a lessening of depression symptoms in groups of patients whose depression had been previously found to be treatment-resistant, which is absolutely bloody fantastic (the results, not the treat-ment-resistant depression). And after now having taken magic mushrooms during many a trip to Amsterdam, I believe the studies to be accurate.

(Disclaimer: magic mushrooms, I know, are not the same as taking psilocybin in a controlled environment and in the pres-ence of a therapist or someone who can handle you if you freak out. I just liked them, OK? Of course, a dosage that makes you see glitter is not the recommended amount to take regularly to help with your mental health. Also, while the treatment sounds exciting, you can guarantee it will affect everyone differently and not work for all of us saddos.)

Psilocybin studies have shown that it 'gently stimulates' the serotonin system in the brain[11] and sort of... relaxes the mind a bit. Those who have taken it often talk about 'seeing things clearly for the first time', and it's widely thought to open up a 'therapeutic window of opportunity' where we're more sus-ceptible to new ways of thinking, and have a clearer perspective when looking at our behaviours. The studies say nothing about the glitter, but I definitely saw that.

Once it gets into your stomach, psilocybin is converted into psilocin, which 'crosses the blood-brain barrier, and then works by exerting partial agonist effects on brain 5-hydroxytryptamine (5-HT) 2A receptors, among others, and can alter normal waking consciousness'.[12] Which, in human language, means that the psilocin binds to the bits in the brain that are ready to receive serotonin, but have likely been waiting for a while if you're depressed. This is essentially the exact opposite function of an SSRI antidepressant, which inhibits serotonin re-uptake. Curious. Psilocybin acts as a widener or opener of the brain, where SSRIs are seen by many as something that blunts our emotions or brain power.

Some people describe a slightly terrifying-sounding 'psychedelic turbulence' after ingesting psilocybin, where they feel like their anxiety is heightened and their body temperature is lowered for thirty to forty-five minutes before the psychedelic bliss. Such are the fantastic-so-far results of psilocybin, though, that the turbulence sounds like a tiny blip on the way to paradise.

One study on twelve volunteers (small, but psilocybin is illegal so these studies have to have a big song and dance about them before they can get anyone to participate... pick me, drug people!) showed that two doses of psilocybin significantly lifted depression for three weeks in all participants, and five of them managed to not have any depressive symptoms for three whole months.

Woah.

fMRI scans of participants' brains after they took psilocybin showed 'resting activity' in the amygdala, which has been shown to play hostess to heightened activity in the brains of those of us with depression. The scans also show 'looser connections' within brain networks that were previously connected pretty solidly. The connections eventually restore themselves, and neuroscientists have likened this to a 'reset' of the brain; it can help you stop your learned, compulsive and negative thought patterns. So, basically, CBT but with less human contact and little boxes, and more sparkles. I'm in.

This is all lovely, but how can I get my hands on some of it?

It's thought that psilocybin could become a prescription medication in the UK within the next three years, but three years is a long, long time if you're in the black hole. Many states within the US, though, actually made psilocybin legal in 2020. Oregon was not just the first US state to legalize psilocybin, but also the first jurisdiction in the world to lay out plans for regulating the drug's therapeutic use, legalizing consumption of psychedelic drugs in regulated, licensed and supervised facilities (expected to come into place in 2023). Then, in June '21 Texas and Connecticut enacted laws allowing medical research into psilocybin as treatment for mental health issues. Although Oregon is not the first place in the US to loosen its legal ropes around psilocybin (cities including Oakland, Denver, Ann Arbor and Washington, DC, voted to effectively decriminalize it), it is the first to put forward a structure that enables research into legal therapeutic use. The main bulk of the research is being focused on post-traumatic stress disorder (PTSD), but this loosening of legal restraints is opening up research into a wider host of mental health gremlins around the world.

In 2021, Compass Pathways (headquartered in the UK) conducted the largest psychedelic drug trial to date. Across twenty-two sites in North America and Europe, 223 participants with Treatment Resistant Depression were given controlled doses of psilocybin. While 223 people might not sound massive for a study, if you imagine them all being in your house at the same time the number suddenly gets quite intense.

In their words, 'We have completed the largest randomized, controlled, double-blind psilocybin therapy study ever done. The topline results show rapid and sustained response for patients receiving a single 25mg dose of COMP360 psilocybin with psychological support.' In my words, everyone was given a single dose of the good stuff, in varying sizes. They all had to taper off their antidepressants before the trial, and participants got a randomized dose of either 25mg, 10mg or 1mg. The 10mg and 1mg people didn't really show a lot of difference (I am hugely summarising here btw), while at least twice the number of participants in the 25mg group were assessed to be in remission for their depression by the third week of the trial, compared with the others.

A much smaller study in the UK (which was also funded by Compass Pathways – we see you, Compass Pathways) set out to analyse simultaneous dosing, i.e. giving a dosage to multiple people at the same time. Potential medications need to be studied like this to determine the safety of scaling up the numbers for further trials, which would replicate the drug being used at scale as a treatment. The more people who test safely, the more likely it is for the drug to be approved.

This study used eighty-nine participants, sixty of whom received the 25mg or 10mg dose, while twenty-nine unfortunate souls were stuck with placebos and acted as the control group. Gutted. Importantly, all participants also received one-to-one support from psychotherapists. They were given their dose in a 'controlled setting', which sounds a bit intense but probably just means 'a safe environment' rather than 'in a dystopian lab with humans strapped to wooden boards and their eyes being pinned open', and then monitored for twelve weeks.

The study concluded that doses from 10 to 25mg of psilocybin can be administered safely to up to six participants at the same time, which although small, is a lovely glint of sunshine breaking through the doom clouds.

What's more, the blurred legal lines (not in the creepy Robin Thicke sense) around the sale of psilocybin in places like Canada and the Netherlands has meant that savvy-sellers and scientists in those areas have been able to further investigate the effects of psilocybin and other mushroom compounds (like Reishi, Chaga, Lion's mane, etc.) on our mental health. Lion's mane, for example, is in the early stages of being proven to be effective at managing attention deficit hyperactivity disorder (ADHD). So it's not just depression that these muddy-tasting shrooms have the power to fix.

So you're telling me to get off my tits every day?

Legally, I have to say I'm not telling you to do that (but honestly you do you, hun). The powerful compounds that people ingest en masse to 'get wrecked' can have a hugely profound effect when taken in microdoses. A microdose is a teeny, weeny, little amount that is not enough to make you feel high, and absolutely nowhere near enough to make you trip and see your dead childhood pet in the sky and cry giant tears of alphabetti spaghetti. It's the dosage that is important here, as 'I'm trying out the effects of microdosing' doesn't really mean 'I'm having shrooms for breakfast every day and I'm always off my tits.'

If psilocybin sounds a bit too intense and perhaps a worrying thing to add to your already boggled mind (and there's not yet enough research around taking it at the same as SSRIs… but it may render them pointless if it's doing the opposite), it's worth noting that some of these mushroom compounds, such as Reishi and Lion's mane, are non-psychedelic and can have very calming effects. I've tried microdosing a few times with Reishi extract, which does not contain psilocybin and is not psychedelic. Reishi extract and Lion's mane (which I haven't tried, but a pal with ADHD and depression has done so and told me, 'All I've had is bad news every day this week and I'm rolling with it all a lot better') are both easily purchasable (you can even get them on Amazon) and fall into the 'medicinal mushroom' category. They've been used in Chinese medicine for years. For me, one microdose of Reishi every three days really took the edge off. The first time I took one I needed a nap quite urgently within about four hours. The second time I felt like I'd had a pint of espresso and was typing with smoke coming outta my fingers. Then it levelled out, and I noticed a difference in my mood. I didn't react so crankily to annoyances at work, and generally felt a lot calmer and more in control.

It's worth mentioning here that psychedelics have been shown to have very low potential for addiction – but anything's possible. There's no scientific evidence that cheese is addictive but a quick glance at my jowls would suggest otherwise. And there are heaps of different mushroom extracts to try, all with differing effects. As with anything, the effects will vary from person to person, and it's all about finding what dosage, frequency and variant works for you. Researching online is helpful, as most merchants in Canada or the Netherlands really know what they're talking about. Personally, I go for the shops that look like a bougie fragrance store rather than the ones called BOB MARLEY 420 RIPPER TRIPPERZZ, but up to you.

It's not only depression that lovely, lovely drugs can help with, though, and it's not just psilocybin that's being tested. Alternative treatments seem to be having a real moment in the scientific world. The scientists over at the University of California, San Francisco, say they're conducting research into the effects of ketamine, LSD and ecstasy along with its related compounds – presumably separately, otherwise that would be… quite a mad sesh.

The NHS in the UK is also looking into experimental drug trials, with studies taking place in Oxford (with ketamine), alongside a veritable ABUNDANCE of new psychedelic research centres being set up by universities and other groups.

CBD (little explainer on that overleaf) has also recently been proven to be Very Fucking Effective Indeed when used topically to treat muscle pain. As we all know, living with chronic pain is of course going to get you in the Speedy Boarding queue to Sad Town, so the fact that there's something so effective to treat muscle pain now is a brilliant start. Most of the products available are unregulated, though, and there's potential for CBD to react with other medications or blood thinners that people might be on, especially if someone is already taking arthritic medicine.

While there are yet (at the time of writing, legal people) to be any CBD products officially legalized for pain use, a combination of CBD and THC (see overleaf) products was legalized by Health Canada, which is where I bought some pain-relief cream for my dad. He says it was 'actually very good, thanks', so I'm not really sure what more research there is to be done.

Wait, slow down, what's up with all these initials?

CBD stands for cannabidiol, which is part of the cannabinoids family. Cannabinoids are found in the *Cannabis sativa plant*. There are more than 480 different compounds present in the plant, and only around sixty-six are categorized as cannabinoids – which are also produced naturally in our bodies (called endocannabinoids, or endogenous cannabinoids).

Our bodies contain endocannabinoid receptors, largely in our central nervous system (CB1 receptors) and peripheral nervous system (CB2 receptors), which welcome along any new endocannabinoids with a friendly hug (or 'binding' if you want to be scientific about it). Everyone produces different levels of endocannabinoids, which makes the whole thing quite hard to test, monitor and regulate.

CBD is also often referred to as 'hemp'. You can buy hemp clothing and paper and stuff, but I'm yet to be convinced as to why you'd want to bother.

Tetrahydrocannabinol (THC) is CBD's drunk aunty. It's also found in cannabis, and is the compound that gets you high. CBD is the chill one, THC is the raver. While I do appreciate THC and have shared many good times with her, I'm sticking to the CBD stuff here.

The location of the receptors on our nervous system is why CBD products can be so effective in pain management or inflammation. CBD's also been touted as a brilliant, soothing pal to bring along to confront your anxiety demons – which is a litttttle contradictory as CBD is not meant to be psychoactive, yet apparently affects your brain in such a way that it soothes anxiety?

It seems to be that the marketing outweighs the research at the moment, as not too many studies have actually been undertaken on the effects of CBD as a treatment for anxiety, and it seems to be anec-data (read: internet hype) showing that, for some, CBD works more effectively than an SSRI. There is a sprinkling of tiny studies that show that CBD reduced symptoms of social anxiety disorders in participants, but the studies are so teeny that I wouldn't feel totally confident in reeling off their findings.

Cannabinoids in general have also been proven to be a bit of a hero ingredient in skincare, but I'm not here to talk about your face, I'm here to talk about what's *inside* your face. Omg, how gross. I mean your brain. Anyway. Let's get back to the shroomy stuff.

Self-actualisation in the abroads

There are now psychedelic retreats emerging in Jamaica and the Netherlands, where you're very much *not* left on your own during or after your dosing experience. These retreats are not offered as a cure for any mental health condition, but are more about 'personal growth'. Synthesis (the institute from the Netherlands I used to make me sound clever earlier on in this chapter) says that its 'psychedelic supported retreats offer participants the potential for personal growth, emotional breakthroughs and spiritual development'.

MyCo Mediations in Jamaica is a little more forward, saying that their 'Psilocybin-assisted therapy can provide an accelerated path to deep healing, new perspectives, connectedness, and feelings of well-being. 91 per cent of our retreat guests consider their experience with psilocybin 'positively life-changing.' Our experience is that this approach to healing may be the path you have been seeking.'Results of data collection pre- and post-retreat at the Synthesis Institute showed that, on average, participants felt a 37-per-cent reduction in depressive feelings compared to the baseline they were at before the retreat. Two weeks later, this had improved to 43 per cent.

Forty-three-per-fucking-cent. That (and let me show off my maths skills here) is feeling almost HALF as depressed as you were before (told you). Half! Those results almost make you (you? Or me?) not care about the potential bad trips or losing control. Honestly if someone told me all I had to do to feel almost HALF as depressed as I currently do is to eat some rank nobbly walnut things before freaking out, dancing naked and masturbating in front of a spiritual guru before vomiting into a ceremonial vase... OK, yes, I admit it does give me *some* pause, but not much.

What is the risk of something like that actually happening while on a guided psilocybin retreat, though? I've spoken to a fair whack of depressed people about their opinion of psychedelics and their potential for improving our mental health, and a notable number of them were really not keen on the idea because of the accompanying potential for it all to go very pear shaped. A lot of folk said that they'd only feel comfortable using psychedelics if they were in a safe space that they knew really well, and were with people they knew and trusted – even when it comes to microdosing. These are psychedelics, right? Psychedelics make you dance like a chicken while crying about your trauma and licking the walls, right?

Not so much.

The retreats have a thorough screening process in place to determine each applicant's suitability for the experience. While they don't claim to diagnose, treat or cure any mental health problems, they certainly don't want anyone to be having a horrible time or to react badly to the doses. Retreat attendees generally receive three 'guided doses' during their week of stay, and are in the presence of experienced 'facilitators' who can look after them. There's a great review of the Jamaican retreat by Decca Aitkenhead in the *Sunday Times*, in which she refers to having had the best days of her life. This is no mean feat for Decca, who is renowned as one of the best interviewers and journalists to ever grace pages with her words – and those words are never minced.

The group that were on the same retreat as Decca all reported feeling significantly altered for the better, once they returned home. Decca herself was surprised when epiphanies came to her in the early hours of the morning, offering simple solutions to problems she previously struggled with.

However, Decca also had a 'nightmare trip' the first time she took a dose of psilocybin. This happens to around a third of the people who attend the retreat, according to MycoMeditations, and is alleged to be 'the purging of the trauma inside you'. Sounds like an absolute NOPE, but the benefits that come afterwards might be worth it.

Let's go back to the published data around the Synthesis retreats. It's important to note here that participants who experienced the most significant decrease in depression bleughness after attending the retreat were those who engaged in psychotherapy in the weeks and months afterwards, and spoke to others who'd been through similar experiences. There's a word for this, and it's called 'integrating' – when you actively make your psychedelic experiences part of your daily life. For those who experienced decreased feelings of depression and anxiety, it was journalling which helped them post-retreat. Alas, this is yet another thing that doesn't just work like a magic silver bullet of joy, but is *something we're going to have to work on* to ensure we get the maximum benefits. Brains are so annoying.

After the four-weeks-post-retreat check-in, the next data collection took place six months after the retreat, and resulted in the average reduction in depressive feelings swinging back to 34 per cent. Does this mean that we're gonna have to schlep over to Amsterdam every six months if we want to keep our mental wellbeing tickety-boo?

Psychedelic practitioners have been quoted as saying that those who have a crack at psilocybin dosing really do need continued aftercare and therapy. Therapy is so spendy it's essentially a luxury item, as we know, so does this put psilocybin out of reach for so many of us and make our health related to our income? The MycoMeditations retreats in Jamaica start at $4,300 for a week. A psilocybin chocolate bar will be over $50, and the truffles are about $2 a gram. (I've tried them all apart from the retreat. Please, someone send me to Jamaica.)

The fact is that this is still such an emerging field, and the studies just aren't there. Legalization for medical research is widening slowly, and hasn't been around long enough to accommodate a study that looks at patients' aftercare needs a year after participating in a psychedelic experiment.

The retreat providers are very clear in their messaging that psilocybin is not a cure for a mental health condition but being offered as a 'tool to assist you in your journey'.

Psilocybin-focused – or 'vacayshrooms' as I personally think they should be known – have been shown to be pretty profoundly effective at revisiting, exploring and dealing with previous emotional trauma. The resulting effect is described as the oft-wielded-in-reality-dating-shows phrase: Emotional Breakthrough. But here it's not described as 'realizing Johnny was a player' and instead as 'facing emotionally challenging events, feelings and past traumas by freely exploring them without resistance', and resulting in participants feeling less anxious following the retreat.

The Synthesis Institute says, 'This is an important finding and supports what other studies in the past years already showed: experiencing an emotional breakthrough seems to be an important factor in explaining the improvement in quality of life observed after a psychedelic experience.'

Of course, there will have been a lot of other factors contributing to participants' increased or decreased mental wellbeing that weren't being measured. Maybe some people got new puppies or had a load of lovely shags. Maybe some people lost loved ones, got divorced or had to spend an evening watching their cat sit on somebody else's lap. The folk at the Synthesis Institute do say that 'these findings should not be interpreted as a suggestion that attending this retreat can serve as a treatment for depression or anxiety, but as a testament to the potential positive impact on a person's overall wellbeing that attending a psychedelic ceremony can have'.

But I've written it all now, so it's staying in.

Obviously, as with anything (except maybe ice cream), there's a possibility it's going to go horribly wrong and not have the dream effects, and drugs work differently with everyone who casts a glance into their glittery portal of joy. Sometimes it turns out to be a slimy, mouldy portal of doom. Sometimes, as with antidepressants, the expectations are just too high.

Life on the internet means that the language being used around psychedelic research is often squished into headlines that insanely sensationalize it, in order to lure us into clicking on the article and giving the publisher 0.02p of revenue from display ads. This means that if you're scrolling through the news, you might see something that says 'Two doses of psilocybin shown to be the same as seven years of therapy, ten Bloody Marys and one good shag'.

In fact, real headlines that actually exist include:

- 'A MAGIC CURE: A single dose of magic mushrooms can treat anxiety and depression'
- 'Half of depression patients given just TWO doses of magic mushroom compound were symptom free a month later'
- 'Just ONE dose of magic mushrooms can ease anxiety and depression for five YEARS in cancer patients'
- 'Magic mushrooms found to heal depression and PTSD'

Advertisements for telemedicine ketamine company Mindbloom even claim it gives you 'five years of therapy in just a few sessions', while prominent figures in the psychedelic space are saying that 'psychedelics are like packing 10,000 hours of psychotherapy into four hours'.

It's true that psilocybin has #blessed a lot of people with its truly incredible benefits, but it's also true that getting mashed on mushrooms is not going to do the same thing to your mind and wellbeing that twenty sessions with a smart therapist will.

Psilocybin retreats and their benefits do sound sensational (if anyone wants to send me to Jamaica to report back, please do so), but they might not change your life in the ways described above. Instead, it's more realistic to think that, if you take a larger dose of psilocybin, you're likely to feel light and happy, and if you take microdoses then you're likely to feel that on a lesser level that keeps you functioning in your daily life.

Of course, the fear of having a bad trip or 'resetting your brain the wrong way' and ruining yourself forever might prevent you from trying any of these treatments, but this can be soooomewhat eliminated if you take a monitored dose of psychedelics with professional guidance and supervision, followed by psychotherapy. There have been incidents reported where some people have had manic episodes after trying out psychedelics, though. If you're just gonna bomb a load of mushrooms and hope for the best, you're on your own and godspeed.

Another psychedelic that's been quietly helping a lot of people is ayahuasca. Ayahuasca (eye-ah-wass-kah) is an Amazonian medicine containing the active ingredient DMT (see overleaf). It's a muddy-tasting (yet again) drink made from the 'prolonged heating or boiling of the *Banisteriopsis caapi* vine (containing the DMT) with the leaves of the *Psychotria viridis* shrub' (which, to be fair, doesn't sound like it'll taste like a Kinder Bueno). DMT is illegal, so ayahuasca retreats are often found masquerading as yoga retreats or 'wellness meditation retreats'.

Hang on, more initials. What are you on about with DMT?

DMT stands for Dimenthyltryptamine and is a strong hallucinogenic drug. It's found naturally in some plants, and isn't used for anything traditionally medical. It's been used in religious ceremonies in South American cultures for years, and seems to exist purely to make us trip balls. Now, its psychedelic effects are being experimented with as a possible solution or treatment for some mental health issues. Very few of these experiments seem to be taking place in medical institutions... more so on beaches and in fields surrounded by people singing 'Kumbaya'.

Ayahuasca is being used as a therapeutic treatment and getting a great reputation for helping to reduce anxiety and stress, but anecdotally it is said to actually be pretty damn awful for depression and can even make it worse. A lot of ayahuasca shamans (the practitioners) won't agree to someone practising with them if they have depression, and a teensy study in 2019 showed that four out of fourteen people in an ayahuasca group were in hospital for over a week following the experiment.

A week.

Two months after the Compass Pathways study ended, twelve of the participants reported suicidal ideation or behaviour. But as this was such a long time after the trial, the Compass folk said it would be unjust to assume those nasties were directly related to participating in a psilocybin study, and could have been from anything, really. The lack of control groups and the inability to

CAN'T YOU TAKE 'SHROOMS FOR THAT NOW, PET?

remove other contributing factors from life really gets in the way of these studies, dunnit?

I have a bodacious friend who I won't out in this book, but who has given me permission (promise) to tell you about their experiences of microdosing LSD, which they started to do after nearly taking their own life one night by jumping off the Clifton Suspension Bridge in Bristol, UK.

No idea why, because I'm terrified of heights, but that was my plan,' she told me. 'But I stopped myself and phoned the Samaritans, and the guy I spoke to was so awful, and not comforting whatsoever, that it kind of jolted me out of this weird state, and I decided, 'Right I'm going to live, at least until tomorrow… so I can complain about you.'

But it was a total wake-up call, and I realized I had to do something, before it consumed me, or killed me, or I did some kind of damage that was irreversible. So I told a few people I was very, very sad indeed (friends, husband), and obviously they knew something wasn't OK so it didn't exactly come as a surprise. I thought about going back to the doctors and asking to go back on anti-depressants, but I was ashamed and felt like I'd failed to live life on my own or something. And it felt like an impossible task.

I'd been recommended a book about microdosing with LSD, called A Really Good Day. I did as much research as I could and bought some very good acid from the dark web. I thought if it didn't work then I would go back to antidepressants, but I just needed to know if there was another option.

It's not for everyone, and obviously there are potential legal implications to taking a class A drug, but it was like someone switched on all the lights in a part of my brain, where before there had been total darkness for a really long time.

For my pal, it sounds like these microdoses had the same effect on them that antidepressants have for so many: clearing the fog. Not fixing anything or removing the darkness completely (because ANNOYINGLY that takes work, ugh), but making everything seem a little lighter and a little easier.

I used the microdosing as a trigger to put more long-term strategies in place. Like meditation, which I do pretty much every day, and trying to practise generally good mental hygiene. Exercise if possible. Take 5-HTP (natural SSRI alternative), drink a lot less booze, and generally be more mindful.

After a few months of microdosing I felt like I wanted to step things up a notch, so I took a large dose of LSD with a friend, and it was like hitting a hard reset on my brain. I felt a surge of overwhelming happiness and had this desire to spend the time figuring some stuff out. I know… It's annoying to hear about other people's trips, but I remember one moment I let go of all this anxiety that I felt like I'd been carrying about myself. About my fear of failing, and of being vulnerable. I confronted it, and cried, and honestly I haven't felt this good for ages. I remember lying there, feeling like I was connected to everything in the universe, rather than sitting outside it as a separate entity, which is just how I'd felt for so long…

82

Now I'll do a 'therapeutic' trip whenever I need a hard reset, which has so far been once in the last six months. It's about as far away from a 'party' trip as you'd imagine. In the last one I meditated alone, watched jellyfish videos, took a long bath, and hiked up a big hill at 5 a.m. so I could go and 'meet the sunrise'. When I got there, I took off my shoes, sat on the grass and looked out across the city and thought... God, I wish I'd known about all this sooner.

Can you take them on antidepressants, though?

Look, people don't want to get sued for giving you the wrong advice, and any institute researching the benefits of psilocybin will likely tell you to 'make sure you check with your medical practitioner before cracking on with the shrooms, yeah?.' The reality is that most medical practitioners have absolutely no fucking idea what cocktail of antidepressants and psilocybin dosages will or won't work for you. The subject and the research is too young to know, and as with every bloody thing related to your mental health, it's usually different for everyone.

Where psilocybin sits on the scale of Legit Western Medicine to Eastern Medicine (or what some people prefer to call 'that woo-woo shit') is still pretty murky. There is research taking place within Western medical practices, but a large number of medical professionals wouldn't consider it part of their practice because it's 'alternative'. Well, there were probably also a few who said, 'Surely poppies can't do anything to you?' and LOOK AT US NOW, MEDICS (I have no idea who I'm talking to here).

The fact is that both psilocybin and most antidepressants work with our serotonergic system, so there is a chance that it could become overstimulated if we're following our fluoxetine with a little mushroom chaser. Because of this, most practitioners will recommend that you don't combine the two as it could lead to serotonin syndrome – a pretty serious drug reaction caused by a high build-up of serotonin in the body. Too much serotonin can make you shiver and shit yourself (well, get diarrhoea, but that didn't fit my alliteration fantasy) or it can give you severe muscle rigidity, fever and seizures. In some cases it can even kill you.

Oh, the irony of trying so hard to be happy and stay alive that you ended up with serotonin syndrome and just big fat died anyway.

So much research is being put into the effects of psilocybin without variables like SSRIs coming into the mix that there simply hasn't been enough work done for me (or anyone; it's not like I'm Mrs Big Wig O' Drugs) to give a solid conclusion about antidepressant and psilocybin combos. There was some research which suggested that SSRIs might lessen the effects of psychedelics, but the researchers are too busy finding out other important stuff about the treatment, which is fair enough really. The findings also vary for SNRIs and MAOIs, and really you should be cautious about what you're putting into your brain if you're thinking of trying a combo. I am not a doctor, I'm just some sad twat with an appetite for experimental practices and the voice of an angel.

If you do want to stop taking antidepressants before you try microdosing, for fuck's sake taper off them properly, you beautiful but sad and irresponsible being.

Sounds lush. How do I put them
IN ME NOW?

First of all, chill. This chapter wasn't meant as a promotional pamphlet, but as more of a rainbow-coloured window into the world of psychedelic research. I massively encourage you to do your own research before dabbling.

That said, there are plenty of places you can buy non-psychedelic mushroom extracts. Most health-food stores stock them, and they're your best bet if you want to go and speak to a human about which one might be the best for you. If you hate speaking to people, do some research online and buy them from the internet.

If you live near or are visiting Canada or the Netherlands, there are heaps of shops with knowledgeable salespeople who can advise on anything from legal mushroom extracts to psilocybin chocolate, THC tinctures, CBD creams and pure psilocybin shrooms.

Of course, you can also just consider yourself a little bit smarter after reading this, and watch with interest as the studies develop. Of course it's up to you. I'll continue to experiment when it feels right, and hopefully land a place on a retreat if anyone wants to pay for me to go to Jamaica? Anyone?*tumbleweed*

The clapbacks

What to say to someone who suggests you get baked on magic mushrooms:

'You know, that's not a bad idea. Got any?'

CHAPTER 4

You should go for a run, mate

Telling a depressed person to try going for a run to feel better is like telling someone to grow a third ear to hear better. We'd love to be able to do it and there's no doubt that it would improve the situation, but we can't. We physically cannot. We mentally cannot. It's not happening. Stoppit.

Alongside 'Oh my cousin's sister went forest bathing once for, like, half an hour, and she's totally cured!', 'Exercise will fix you y'know' is one of the first merry quips people will make upon hearing that you're playing host to the demons in your head.

God, I'd love to be one of those people on American dramas who go for long, transformative runs whenever they need to pound out a problem. The president's safety could be at risk and the person threatening them is your husband? Go for a run. An assassination attempt has been made on your boss, and you think you might know who did it? Go for a run. Your child has been taken by a Russian sex-slavery gang? Go for a run. Off they always run, the brooding heroes. They're the type who can run in any weather and can fit into a montage of gorgeous, iconic scenery as they run for miles and miles. By the end of the run, they always know what to do.

It's a bit of a big leap to become an inspirational running montage when you're spending your fourth hour in total darkness in a bed that you've soaked through with your tears, though.

The worst thing about it is that we KNOW exercise will help, right? We know it, we honestly do, and that's what adds to the shame of not being able to really sit up in bed, let alone voluntarily *leave* the bed, the bedroom, the flat, and then to *move around at a faster pace*. Are you high? We can't do that, we're stuck. Telling a depressed person to try going for a run generally makes the depressed person feel ashamed for not actually having been for a run. They'll feel guilty for not actively seeking out a known aid to mental health problems. They'll feel like a failure after being reminded that they're unable to do something to help themselves.

Reminder: if you are this person feeling like a failure, you're absolutely NOT a failure. You're depressed. Depression has messed up your head and your energy and all your limbs and honestly well done to you if you're not just flailing about and screaming WHYYYY? into the void. I applaud you.

The thing about the 'exercise makes you better' advice is that it's mostly coming from a good place, and often it comes from people who have experienced depression themselves and found that exercise has helped them clear out the dusty demons from their head. But in order to exercise, you really need to be out of the worst, darkest, heaviest and most bed-bound part of depression. You at least need to be at a stage where you can get dressed and pretend to function most days. I couldn't have got to that stage without the help of my medication. It takes a while for the real exercise endorphins to kick in – even the people of the great un-depressed find that to be the case, and someone feeling the good stuff might find it hard to remember just how dark the darkness was beforehand. Like when you just remember the beautiful beach holiday, and not the two eleven-hour flights it took to get there plus the eight-hour layover where you sat next to a man with a noisy chicken.

Failure to launch

Depression makes you think that most things are impossible, and if not impossible, then definitely hopeless. Depression convinces you that there's no way you can leave the house or go downstairs, or leave your bed, or even sit up. Depression has injected a thick treacle of gloom into your brain that's very cleverly convinced you that you're nothing, and nothing you do will mean anything, and that there's no point even trying.

During the absolute bottom-of-the-chasm periods, turning on the bedside lamp seems like a monstrous task that should really be in the Olympics or something. This is *turning on the lamp*, never mind donning a sports bra and trotting out for a jog around the block. This usually leads to some fairly extreme feelings of guilt that you're not doing more to try to combat how you're feeling, and can leave you questioning if you're dwelling in your misery. Are you making it worse for yourself when you should be actively trying to heal your body through the apparently spiritual and beautiful ritual of going for a jog?

This continues in a vicious circle and, quite obviously, doesn't help you feel better at all. I get it.

When people told me to go for a run while I was very much wading through darkness, it often ended up just being a reminder that my body and I were failing to complete pretty basic functions – as well as often coming across as a flippant dismissal of the severity of depression by suggesting that a few minutes of light endorphins will sort me out, mate. When it's suggested in a very light and casual way, it feels like a suggestion of a very simple, basic task, that everyone else can do apart from you. 'Shall we have another coffee? Do you think you should start running?'

Not to dismiss the real benefits of exercise when someone is able to do it; pushing your body to a limit that you don't think you can handle is oddly satisfying. Sure, there are times during a run or a class when you might feel like you're going to vomit, and that's never fun, but at vomit o'clock your mind is purely thinking, 'Oh God, am I gonna throw up all over myself?' and not, 'I want to die.' Exercise engages your whole body and forces your brain to think differently. Exercise is as much for the mental benefits as it is for the physical, and hurting yourself to improve yourself gives you a feeling of achievement, which is such a welcome break from the constant feelings of gloom. But the lighthearted 'advice' from people suggesting you hit the gym can feel like you've already done a boxing class and been punched straight in the stomach.

When you've had to cancel all your weekend plans because you can't bring yourself to get out of your bed, or when you've had to call in sick to work because the thought of facing another human being makes your stomach fill with lead and your heart feel like it's going to explode, or when you told yourself you'd schlep out of the house this week and go for a wholesome walk with a lovely podcast but the reality is you're sitting in the dark staring at the wall and suddenly four hours have gone by and your face is wet with tears... are you really gonna go for a quick run?

Sitting up in bed is a monstrous effort. Leaving the bed seems like climbing Everest. Going any further than the bathroom – well, that's just asking someone to take a long walk off a short plank. No thanks, back to bed we go.

Do not feel bad (easier said than done, I know). If someone has never suffered from depression themselves, they are unlikely to understand what you're going through. Hey! Why not wing them a copy of this fine book? When I was at my absolute worst, I couldn't understand how people could leave the house. Similarly, these non-depressed people do not understand that sometimes you don't even piss all day because getting out of bed and going to another room is a momentous and enormous task.

I cannot stress enough that this does not involve pissing the bed. Just festering in bed. A piss-free bed.

The main thing that needs to be done before any kind of exercise can even be thought about is getting out of bed. This sounds fairly simple in the grand scheme of movements, but as you know, it's near impossible when you're sinking.

Couch surfing

I started, eventually, with the baby step of getting out of bed and moving to the sofa – which ended up happening for the simplest reason: I needed to wash the bedsheets. The sheet underneath me was feeling rough on my skin and the pillows were caked in mascara, tears and dribble. Probably snot too, as I'm being so honest with you. The entire bed area was starting to smell a little questionable, and I felt pretty disgusted with myself, so I slugged out of bed and started taking off the bedclothes. The exact details of these few minutes aren't crystal clear, but I'm pretty sure I took the sheets to the machine and beyond the washing machine, I saw the sofa. The sofa looked comfier than sorting out laundry, so I schlepped over to it and flopped on. It was quite nice on the sofa. I could see out the window, which felt more productive than lying down and not seeing out the window. I went back the next day. And the next.

This was after a long time of choosing the bed option. Still with a duvet, in the darkness, and largely asleep or crying, but sometimes I would have the curtains open and be able to see the outside. Major growth. Huge.

Depression saps your energy from you to the point where anything other than going back to sleep just uses up too much of what little strength you have. This doesn't exactly bode well for signing up to a course of healing aqua-biking.

Emotional energy is hugely important. If you're depressed and drink seven cans of Red Bull, chances are you're still going to want to lie in the dark, unmoving. The Latin derivative for emotion is *emotere*, which literally translates to 'energy in motion'. Emotional energy can be described as the feeling of our emotions running through us; if you're happy and celebrating, you're likely to be in 'high spirits' and thus high energy. If you're sad and crying or staring at a wall, you'll probably be quite up for a nap. One of the biggest symptoms of depression is low energy and fatigue, and sleeping all the time. The emotional part of our brain (the amygdala) affects everything else in the brain, and if our emotions are in the crapper then it's going to be very difficult indeed to be motivated physically.

You need to be at a certain point of feeling even the teeniest ounce of motivation to consider any exercise at all, and running is hardly gonna be first on the list.

When we're depressed, though, it's pretty tricky to tap into any of our positive emotions. A depressed mind is fizzing over with guilt and shame, fear, sadness, apathy and maybe even anger. When we're so tuned into these emotions, we won't have the resources to motivate ourselves. Having plenty of sleep and a healthy breakfast with a vitamin smoothie will do diddly squat if your mind is dark, and you'll need to change your emotional energy – but for the love of God HOW?

It's tricky and involves a lot of internal arguments and forcing yourself to do stuff, which nobody likes. Sorry. But also, it's no fun constantly crying and yearning for darkness, so I guess we have to pick our battles. Before I was engulfed by depression's quicksand I used to find joy in the outdoors. Not doing a hike or anything wholesome, mainly sitting in the park with some crisps, but greenery generally corresponded with relatively good moods for me. Or maybe it's music; whether it's a George Michael bop, a Celine Dion power ballad or a simple melody from Slipknot. When I was at my darkest, though, my formerly favourite things became oppressive. I would close the curtains on a blue sky because it would make me feel even more shame for wanting to lie in the dark instead of frolic in a meadow. I would try my favourite albums and shut them off, too, because it was shameful to feel numbness in place of joy.

According to psychotherapist John-Paul Davies, 'The difficulty is that, when we're depressed, we have little access to these emotions. We'll mainly do things – or stop doing things – out of fear, shame, guilt, anger, apathy or boredom. We lack the emotional energy needed to do anything that might bring the "motivator emotions" more into life.'

That's quite a mouthful if you need a response to someone who's nonchalantly suggesting you sign up for a 10k next week, but you can always refer to the scientific fact that depression quite literally sucks the energy out of you. It's nothing to do with laziness; your brain doesn't have the access to the emotional resource to help you spring out of bed and into your trainers.

A lot of Making Depression a Bit More Tolerable is about forcing yourself to do stuff you really don't want to do, because it'll probably help you eventually. Like a huge, life-threatening, emotionally draining, work- and relationship-affecting tax return.

Starting small is the key. There is no way that one day you're just going to wake up, spring out of bed and into some Instagram-ready workout gear to head off for a rejuvenating run through flower-filled meadows. Sorry to break it to you. But, BUT, maybe you could try to point your toes.

Seriously, try it. If you're sitting, lying, whatever. Extend a leg just a little bit and point your toes really far forward like a ballet dancer, then curl them around the top of your foot as if you're scrunching them into an odd little foot-fist. Hold it as tight as you can for five seconds. Let go. Then pull your toes back towards your shins as far as they will go (not using your hands) and stick your heel out. Hold for five seconds. Stop. Try it with the other foot.

Pretty nice, hey?

When I say I started slow, I mean I started glacially. Small nano-stretches like this can be done from bed or the sofa, and I found that really stretching to the point of a bit of pain actually feels quite good. If you can get anything to click or crunch, even better. It wasn't like I'd do a series of stretches all at once like a bendy Californian, but the stretches did start to make an appearance into my life of darkness, and they felt satisfying. Finally. Something felt something.

So then, that was that for a while, I think maybe around a month or so – time is fairly meaningless when you don't care about its passing. Staying in bed. Sometimes on the sofa. Stretching out the crunchy body of a crone haggard before her time.

I kept stretching, in a way akin to Uma Thurman trying to wiggle her big toe in the Pussy Wagon of *Kill Bill*. I didn't even really do it all that consciously before I started googling 'stretches for a stiff back/sore legs/tight shoulders', etc. Laying down in misery all day doesn't half give you stiff muscles, and it seemingly had got to a point where I wanted to do something about them. Self-care gurus eat THAT.

Of course, lying down in the dark with the brightness on my phone turned all the way down as I stared into it from two inches away from my nose, I noticed that the stretches on the Google results page mostly needed me to at least sit up to actually do them. I probably googled them every day for a week or so, and just scrolled through as if looking at them would somehow transfer their benefits onto me as if I'd done them.

Then, goddammit, I sat up.

I think by that stage I'd got so fed up with myself that I was trying to give myself a shake and a telling-off – telling myself to get a grip and stop procrastinating and to give this stretching lark a go.

Please, stop applauding, honestly. It's fine. Shh. Enough with the cheering.

It's important to note that there was nothing else going on in the way of productivity, here. I was 'working from home' a lot of the time, and not doing much work apart from giving a sad bottle of Campo Viejo a good seeing to. (I mean drinking it, not masturbating with it – I hope this much is clear.) But the stretching was feeling good.

Probably as a combination of both 'oh, this feels... not horrible' and just pure procrastination, I started to google 'yoga for bad backs' (an action I thought made me essentially 103 years old until Covid-19 lockdown turned us all into wizened, crotchety bags of knots) and 'yoga for tight hips' (sexy). I didn't actually do any of the yoga for a while, God no, I just watched the videos before eventually trying to do it myself.

Maybe it took two weeks of watching others do the yogic stretching I thought I should be doing before I 'for God's sake'-ed myself and tried it too.

Annoying, isn't it? There isn't a step-by-step plan to follow to get you from the pits of your dark, unwashed, cold and clammy, sweaty and breathy despair and off to do a sun salutation – and I want to reiterate here that I was still feeling utterly, truly miserable. But stretching out my body made me feel like I'd achieved something, and the tiny stretches I was giving my cramped up, bed-ridden muscles were pretty heavenly – I figured the bigger the stretch might result in the bigger reward, and I was right. Stretching your body is a wonderful release, and we hold so much tension and stress in our muscles. Every time a bone crunched or I touched a toe, it felt like some of my mental pain was being alleviated by this oddly pleasurable physical pain.

Thanks to the world of the internet and people who want to have their faces on it, there's loads of free yoga to try on YouTube. I went for *Yoga with Adrienne* because she has so many super-short sequences for specific stretches or 'issues', as well as the most enormous fluffy dog who sometimes comes to join in.

She is quite perky and cheerful, though, which is annoying.

Nama-stay in bed

When I stopped stretching on my own and started doing yoga under instruction (albeit remote, pre-recorded, sometimes overly enthusiastic American instruction), I was also introduced to a pretty obvious-sounding concept that actually really helped my brain clear a little bit of fog. Breathing.

I KNOW, RIGHT? Breathing. Revolutionary.

But much like I found satisfaction in the painful stretches of my flump-like muscles, yogic breathing is really fucking weird, and gives you another kind of satisfaction when you stretch and empty your lungs to an almost painful point either side. If you've ever done yoga or watched a yoga video, you'll know that the instructors are constantly telling you to 'connect to your breath' and 'breathe into the stretch' – which initially I thought was a load of tosh and just ignored in favour of trying to get on with the actual stretches themselves. But, spoiler alert, when you follow the instructions then you can get the desired result. Turns out that yogic breathing is actually the foundation of yoga, and that doing it when you're not even doing the physical movement is quite beneficial. It basically goes like this:

1. Sit down, cross your legs and remember that you have an abdomen, a diaphragm and a chest. Think about those three things for a sec.
2. Take a deep breath in, through your nose, and keep going. Breathe in slowly, as if you're filling your lungs with as much air as they can carry. Expand your belly, ribcage and chest. Basically 'present' like a male gorilla about to get his rocks off.
3. Hold that breath for a few seconds.

4. Slowly – slllowwllly – release the breath out through your mouth so you feel like you've got nothing left inside you and your lungs are wee prunes. The slowness is important; don't just exhale out in a quick-shot rush as if you just held your breath in a tunnel and you're eleven years old. Control it.

Man, that sounds pretentious, doesn't it? – but it works when you're not doing yoga because it helps focus your mind on something other than doom, thus changing your emotional energy. It works when you are doing yoga, too, as when you exhale you can move into a deeper stretch, and the breathing can help you push your body further than before. It essentially feels like some kind of mild punishment, which you feel you deserve as a depressed glib, so you push into the pain a bit more.

So I stayed in that kind of hopscotch routine for a while. Staying at home, doing some yoga from a video sometimes. Probably getting it all wrong but feeling better after I did it than I had felt before I started it. Also, it's a way to make time push on without really feeling it because you're so busy trying to stretch something that sounded pretty easy but actually has made you feel like you're made of stone.

I didn't expect anything was going to change as a result of my groundbreaking 'staying at home and being sad and sometimes doing a fifteen-minute yoga video' way of life, and it took me a while to notice that anything had changed at all. I was still miserable – but I was a bit less miserable than before. I was still spending my time as a hermit, but it didn't feel quite as heavy. I changed nothing else about my days other than doing some YouTube videos, and it feels a bit sheepish to say, but it got to the point where (possibly thanks to being on medication) I began to care if I was actually doing it right.

Not being the type to have a home studio with enormous mirrors, I had no idea if what I was doing when Adrienne told me to 'lengthen through my spine' or 'firm my outer arms in' or 'close my eyes' was correct; I just did it in a way that felt nice. The only way of seeing if I was actually doing it right would be to go out into the world and get a qualified instructor to show me how I was actually doing it wrong. Um, no thanks.

But the stretching was beneficial, and made me feel productive. Even if before and after I was sitting or lying down and not doing much, the stretches and the fact that I was following someone else's instruction made me feel like I'd achieved something. If I was getting bits wrong at home, would it feel even better if I was shown how to do them correctly? An alarming thought, but yoga can make you feel a little strange (i.e. not miserable) after you've done some, and I was entertaining bold thoughts about maybe one day joining a class. Maybe.

Googling local yoga classes became an interesting new way to procrastinate. Most of them had an 'intro week' offer where you could do 'as many classes as you want!' (calm down) for the week for about £30. I clicked around these websites and left the tabs open for about two weeks before I decided to do anything about it, but if our open tabs represent what's on our mind, the open yoga classes options were sitting at the back of mine as I clumsily flopped around my living room for a few more weeks.

The turning point came when I read Matt Haig's excellent book *Reasons to Stay Alive*, in which he and many anonymous crowdsourced individuals heralded the benefits that yoga gave them and how it helped support their wobbly mental health. People repeatedly listed yoga as one of the things actually keeping them alive, and that's certainly not to be sniffed at. I revisited my open tabs and just went for it. What a wild child.

I signed up to a class that involved everything being booked online, no speaking to a human required, and scheduled in an actual real-life yoga class for that week. Fuck, I had accidentally become Gwyneth Paltrow. Namaste, my children. Pop a jade egg in your vagina and enjoy this organic kale.

With nothing in my vagina, I made my way to the class. I'd booked a 'hot' yoga class because it was freezing in my living room when I was on my laptop, and I desperately wanted to feel warm. Well, 38°C inside will certainly help with that.

'Hello, I'm new and I'm probably going to die,' I said to the instructor as he glided into the room, nose rings glistening and muscles… well, also glistening tbh.

'Just stay in the room,' he said. 'Don't worry about doing everything, because it'll be too hard. Just stay here even if you feel like you might faint. Have a teeny tiny sip of water. If you feel like you want to leave, sit down slowly. Get used to the temperature. It's going to be difficult. Don't let me see you leaving.'

What fun.

Turns out, though, that a fair amount of yoga is about lying down and breathing, which every depressed person alive is already highly skilled at. At the beginning of the session we'd lie on our mats in the hot, humid room, and there would be a few minutes where I either imagined I was in the Bahamas, or I was warm and asleep. Both great options in comparison to bedroom-doom-darkness. After that, the poses were slow, and the instructor would walk among us all as we flamingoe-d on one leg, gently pushing our shoulders or hips or whatever bones we have into the right place.

The thing about yoga is that you can make it as tricky as you want, and you don't reeeeally have to try if you can't be arsed. The teachers always talk about 'pushing into something as much as you feel able to', and if you can't, then you can't, and nobody gets off their mat and marches over to you, points and says HA, LOOK AT YOU, YOU INFLEXIBLE BITCH. Everyone just gets on with it.

So I could try as much as I wanted, and not bother when I wanted, and try to get used to the way the teacher kept asking us to place our hands 'just above your pubic bone' with absolutely no success.

At the end of yoga you also get to lie down for a while again, so that's pretty good, but the thing I was most surprised about was the breathing. Getting into a rhythm of deep breathing for an hour is a little like getting mildly high – especially in a very hot studio.

I'm aware this'll sound a bit 'woo-woo' but breathing into the painful parts of your body as you try to stretch them out and test their limits does a very good job of distracting your brain from the darkness. Even though you're focusing on a different kind of pain that's more immediate, more physical and more cause-and-effect, it's better than the constant pain of really feeling your depression.

Sweating! It's like crying! But with your whole body!

At the end of the class, you're soaked in sweat. It's disgusting, it's like you've taken a shower in your own filthy perspiration. Even my hair was sweating. Some people chose to leave the studio immediately and head off (for which they were very harshly judged in my mind, stinkers); others opted for a hot shower instead. But here's the thing about being covered in sweat: it's gross, yeah, but it's also a sign that you've worked for something. You've pushed yourself and achieved something physical that months ago you would have laughed at. Well, maybe shrugged at, if you had the energy.

The shower afterwards feels like a reward, and you can actually feel it. The sweat and the aches make you feel accomplished; you're not having cold sweats in your bed and aching limbs from tiredness, you're having hot sweat and muscle cramps because you *made your body do something*, and it feels… it feels good? For me it felt a damn sight better than bed-festering did, anyway, and a lot of it was to do with the fact that I'd somewhat defrosted from a state of numbness.

Yoga is slow. It's silent. It's totally at your own pace, and there are no countdown clocks or personal bests to be had. It was the perfect way for me to oh-so-slowly get off my arse and dip a sweaty toe (soz for the visual) into this world of 'exercise' people keep talking about.

Yes, OK, I know I sound dumb again, but the slow, controlled breathing really does relax you, and when you have to breathe in time to your body movements and 'push your breath into your shoulders' – it does actually feel soothing, and fuck knows I needed to be soothed.

Feeling soothed or mildly high *could* be those pesky endorphins that fitness-types seem to have loads of. I'll take that. To be realistic, in a brain and body that is currently programmed to feel nothing but eternal gloom, feeling anything *but* the eternal gloom is like having a bag of MDMA, some blue Smarties and a Lemon Fanta. I imagine.

But here's the thing: our brains are a bit like a huge maze made up of loads of footpaths. The paths form when we have experienced something. Thus, some of the paths are really well trodden as they've been formed by things we do every day, like going to work, getting dressed, speaking English and listening to that new Gaga song again. Some paths started to form and then went nowhere, like when we stopped playing piano when we were fourteen.

When we have new experiences or try to learn new things OR take part in some physical activity, very light, new paths form in our brain maze. The more we do these things, the deeper the paths, and the more natural they become to us. Doing physical activity makes a direct, positive impact on your brain's structure and functioning. We know this. But how much do we realize that the structural changes can lessen the depressive parts of our brain?

Studies have shown that people with depression have a smaller hippocampus,[13] which is a teeny but significant part of our brain that is squished right into the middle of everything. Alas, it looks nothing like a camp hippo, but instead more like cheesy puff (people say it looks like a seahorse but I can't see it).

It's responsible for regulating emotion, memory, learning and motivation. All the things that seem to go totally wonky when we're depressed. The hippocampus also hosts a lot of our 'executive functioning', which I like to think of as a judging panel (like on *The X Factor*) in a boardroom, (like the early seasons) making decisions about how our big dumb body goes about its life.

The decisions they're given are all to do with:

1. Situations that involve planning or decision making
2. Situations that involve error correction or trouble shooting
3. Situations where responses are not well rehearsed or contain novel sequences of actions
4. Dangerous or technically difficult situations
5. Situations that require overcoming strong habitual response or resisting temptation[14]

So the ol' hippocampus and its judging panel have a lot on their plate. However, in the brains of people with depression, the size of the hippocampus has been shown to be smaller, as in, it shrinks in the brains of people who are suffering with depression. Studies have shown that the more depressive episodes a person has, the smaller their hippocampus is likely to be.[15]

Following the study, Professor Ian Hickie from the Brain and Mind Centre said that 'recurrent or persistent depression does more harm to the hippocampus the more you leave it untreated. This largely settles the question of what comes first: the smaller hippocampus or the depression? The damage to the brain comes from recurrent illness.'

There are similar studies that conclude sexual arousal causes neurogenesis in the hippocampus. As in, it regenerates and feels alive. I do wonder if this is why you get so horny when you're suffering a terrible hangover but couldn't find any legit studies to back that up (quite rightly, I suppose, medical research funding is being spent elsewhere).

As a part of the hippocampus is responsible for our 'spatial memories' (e.g. learning routes, places, etc.) I'm chalking this up to be the reason I tried to freeze a tray of water-to-become-ice-cubes in the microwave last week.

So anyway, the more neural pathways we have, the stronger our brains are, and the better functioning our hippocampus can be. Hurrah.

Exercise has been shown to help increase the size of the hippocampus,[16] which means all of us Sad Susans do actually have a chance at making reasonable decisions and generally taking an active role in our own lives, and all the non-depressed people ARE JUST CHEATING. OK, they're not cheating, but they can shine their brain up to have a nice, giant hippocampus that would certainly win first prize at the village fête. Bastards.

Remember, this is a long game so don't try to change everything all at once. Repeatedly replacing your old behaviour with new behaviour will create strong new neural pathways in your brain so that it can become a new habit – it takes an average of sixty-six days to form a new habit so there's no reason to feel like a failure if you don't immediately find yourself going to rooftop dawn yoga every morning.

OK, enough brain science chat for a bit.

So I went back to yoga again. Obviously, I sucked. I could barely do any of the stretches without the squidgy bits of me that should have been muscle twitching uncontrollably. I had to sit down and 'stay in the room' a lot, and sometimes when we were mid-stretch and the teacher asked us to just casually extend something else, it made me fall over. But the sweaty satisfaction was worth it. Also, going to a fifty-five-minute class takes two hours out of your day with the travel and the showering, and that's two sweet hours where you don't have to speak to anyone. Marvellous.

Also, I found the class to be better than the YouTube videos because there's someone talking you through it in real life and you pretty much need to do what they tell you. In a studio, it's much more difficult to just turn off the teacher and go and have a biscuit.

It's a bit spendy, though, and even though I love it, I did start thinking about exercise I could do for free… like running.

PLEASE DON'T CLOSE THE BOOK

I *thought* about running for ages. Probably about five months, at least, and it was when I wasn't in the absolute gloomiest gloom state of depression and was already getting up and about for things, and just silently wanting to die.

I was taking a lot of little trips to try to make myself feel feelings, and I brought along some exercise clothes for running, in my bag, everywhere I went. I lived in stabby North London next to lots of gross roads, so had already ruled out in my head running near home. But going to stay with family or going away on my own meant that there would be beautiful scenery and landscapes fit for the perfect debut transformational running montage. So I thought.

My running gear stayed in my bag, in the same spot, for five months. Always brought with the best intentions, never, ever used.

Baby, I wasn't born to run

One day on one of these 'please feel a feeling' trips, I found myself near to a long, beautiful river, with nothing else to do. It was pretty sunny but not annoyingly sunny, the river looked blue, and there weren't too many people around to get annoyed with.

I went to my Airbnb and put on my running gear for the first time ever. I then pottered about the flat for about two hours, finding things to do that meant I wouldn't need to go for a run. Oh, I should send this email! Oh, I've had a snack so should really let that settle! Oh, I need to look at Instagram for twenty minutes! UGH, STOPPIT. Just go and try it, I thought.

I had downloaded the Nike Run Club app on recommendation from a pal, after I complained about having listened to the Couch to 5k app before (on a couch) and its 'elevator music' making me even more suicidal than usual. The Nike app lets you put your own music on, and a coach talks you through everything as you go.

I chose the Absolute First Time Basic Beginners First Ever Super-Slow Run for Non-Runners Ever in the World from the list, put my headphones in and walked over to the river. I got to the river, I pressed the play button and I tried to do what the nice man in my ears was telling me to do. He had some decent chat and was talking about how I should be feeling and what I should be doing at each part of the twenty-minute session.

Twenty minutes – I know. There was no way I was going to finish it. But (I promise I don't do PR for this app but if anyone from their comms team is reading this then hit me up) the app-man's mixture of chit-chat and cheesy but effective motivation combined with my sophisticated playlist (Emo Bangers 2003) meant that somehow I got to the end of the workout.

I'd done it. A run. A twenty-minute run. I felt like I was going to die (yay!) but also very, very elated. I never thought I would be able to run, but trudging along suuuuper-slowly and listening to Coach Taylor Logan Chad Brad, or whatever his name was, actually made me get there.

I did that same beginner's session about eight times before I moved on to the session called So Now It's Your Second Run or whatever, which is an entire three minutes longer. Would strongly recommend it.

Jogging is a funny one; it essentially replicates the physical symptoms of an anxiety attack, but because you're in control, it makes you feel much calmer. When I run I am a sweating, breathy mess; my heart is pummelling into my chest like a boxer trapped in a suitcase, the pounding surging up to my head. My breathing is fast and hot, and my eyebrows are clogging with sweat – but in an oddly good way after the first ten minutes of hell. The first ten minutes are always hell.

Running hurts. It hurts your lungs, your legs and sometimes your chest. Being in control of pain is pretty satisfying, and underneath it all it's healthy to go for a jog, so the pain is for the greater good.

This is not to say that I am now 'a runner' – I haven't been for about six months as I write this, because I'm always finding excuses not to go. I always, always hate the first ten minutes, but then something clicks and it feels OK – and I've never regretted going for a run. If anything you can just use the excuse to be a run-wanker and drop the 'Oh sorry, I didn't see that, I was out for a ruuuuuun' into a conversation.

It doesn't have to be running – although that might sound a bit obvious. Cardio exercise of all sorts has been proven to particularly annoy the depression demons. A lot of people enjoy going to a class because you just do what you're told and don't have to think. Arranging to do something with a friend makes you less likely to cop out, and it could just be walking. Walking is brilliant.

There's also something really very soothing about being outside and among some kind of greenery. Hard to find in stabby North London, yes, but there are parks you can get to on the bus in order to frolic about. It's actually been scientifically proven that nature and green spaces helps to ease symptoms of painful mental health. Even ol' Flozza Nightingale wrote in 1859 that her patients had the 'most acute suffering when they could not see out of the window'. [17] So there.

'Nature Accessibility' and 'Nature Exposure from Home' have both been shown to have positive effects on depression, anxiety and stress,[18] and there's heaps of evidence to show that spending time in natural, greener environments can improve your mental health.

It doesn't have to be running to get you outside, though. Walking, wheeling or even getting on a nice bus route that goes past some lovely things can be good – or, just stay in and get some plants. I'm serious. The absence of a bank balance allowing for a second home in Vancouver means that a lot of us in teeny flats in urban areas will just have to make do, and plants have been proven to help mental health. It's science.[19] You can argue with me all you like, but you can't argue with science.

The clapbacks

When someone just makes an off-the-cuff comment about exercise that you should do and makes you feel like a big pile of steaming failure... what to say?

'The thing is, depression completely sucks up all your energy – emotional and physical – and it'll take some time for me to get to a place where I'm motivated enough to put my trainers on. I'm aware of the benefits, though, and will be trying it out when I can.'

'I know it will, but I really don't know where to start. Can we arrange to go for a walk next week, please, and don't let me back out of it?'

'Good idea. I'll start now.' (Then you run away.)

CHAPTER 5

Just stay off Instagram for a bit, hun

Social media can be both hugely triggering and immensely soothing when you have a mental health problem, depending on how you use it. Obviously, there are many who are quick to say that social media is a damaging, satanic hell-hole and every scroll on Twitter or Instagram deletes 100 more brain cells as you absorb vapid internet culture, but hold up – this is really not the case.

Yes, there are some aspects of social media that the world would be better without (hello, Kardashians advertising slimming lollipops and people from school posting endless videos of their ugly children). Nobody likes seeing everybody post Aspirational Picnics featuring the entire dip section of Waitrose while they're lying on a pillowcase of their own tears and mascara – but hey, nobody actually *has* to look at them, either.

It's so easy to feel guilty for unfollowing social accounts – particularly those of people you know personally – but really, if their posts make you feel like your life isn't good enough, then hit that unfollow button, honey. Also there is the joy of MUTE on most platforms, which I would highly recommend if you're not feeling brave enough to go full-hog (but honestly people really won't notice if you unfollow them if they're too busy making sure they have the perfect Insta-ready shot of their halloumi fries).

The Royal Society for Public Health did a huge study which indicated that Instagram is *the* most detrimental social platform for our mental health,[20] yet we continue to scroll through it and fall into Insta-story holes and – lo! – post stuff to the platform ourselves.

Other studies have concluded that the more social platforms we use, the more anxious and depressed we're likely to feel.[21] I think I read that on Twitter... or was it Facebook?

It doesn't have to be this way. As definitively as there was room for Leo on the *Titanic*'s door in the sea, there is a way to use social media to – gasp – positively help your mental wellbeing. Look, you might as well give it a go, right? Have you put this fine book down to look at Instagram since you started this chapter? Thought as much (don't worry, I've done it too).

Instagram can actually make you feel validated in a really wonderful way, if you just use it correctly – and yes, this does mean unfollowing Jen from uni who's now a bendy yoga teacher and living in the Cayman Islands, and probably putting a mute on your old boss who made you feel like shite every day and is now off spending her hundreds of thousands of pounds on a seventh house.

Although when you use Instagram you're generally alone (or have just given up on conversation with those around you) and silent, it can feel like a crowded and noisy space. The global access, wide content variety and diverse userbase means that there are always new posts and always a conversation being had that you might want to join. Yes, social media is a toxic little savage that makes us feel alone and friend-less and like our lives aren't as good as they should be and our brunches aren't as pretty as Chloe's from school, but it also gives us access to a load of really fun communities that we might not otherwise ever get to chat to.

Instagram, Snapchat and Twitter all have the creepy ability to connect us to anywhere in the world within three flicks of our thumb. You can search via map, hashtag or location pin and suddenly see exactly what's happening in a drag bar in East London, in an art gallery in New York or on a beach in Brazil. This capacity for global connection has the potential to bring you so much joy, I promise.

Imagine growing up in a rural town with no real action, and feeling unconnected to everything you wanted to experience in the world. No art, no real culture and absolutely no drag queen brunches on a Sunday. No musicians or performers ever come to your town. No rallies ever take place in your city centre, and absolutely nothing ever happens in Borington-on-Trent where you will remain static for the foreseeable future.

Enter Instagram, arriving to show you the world from in between your thumbs. Someone who's completely stuck is able to reach a community on social media – Instagram in particular – and connect with people who they would never have had the opportunity to speak to if it weren't for us all being scrolly-Susans. Whether you're following a body positivity movement like #effyourbeautystandards, a global movement like #timesup or an interior decoration tag like #styleitdark, social media now has a way of keeping you plugged in to almost any community you're interested in.

For what it's worth, I strongly recommend following the #miniaturedaschund tag.

I've found Instagram more interesting by purely unfollowing people who make me feel jealous/underachieving/generally like crap, and instead proactively following a shitload of meme accounts and genuinely hilarious people who actually make me laugh out loud – which is madness when you consider that a great portion of my day is spent fantasizing about never having been born. But if I can find joy there, SO CAN YOU.

Some accounts and hashtags that make me feel joyous

@mkik808 – Mark Kanemura, a choreographer and performer in LA who dedicates every Friday to Carly Rae Jepsen's 'Cut to the Feeling' and uses Instagram to stage daily performances in a variety of wigs and #lewks.

#effyourbeautystandards – a powerful body-acceptance movement that celebrates diverse body shapes and colours, a far cry from promoting a Jessica Rabbit-esque figure and instead rejoicing in living a full life.

@reductress – satirical site taking the absolute piss out of traditional 'women's media', women's issues and female relationships. Recent post: '*4 Christmas dresses that say "I've never had a dick in my mouth.*"'

#**dalmatianpuppy** – obviously.

@**greenmatters** – posting GOOD news about the environment and climate change, highlighting what positive differences are being made. An excellent tonic to the alarming WE'RE ALL GOING TO BURN headlines.

@**jvn** – Jonathan Van Ness is an absolute joy, encouraging us all to look after ourselves and see the positive. He also shares his figure-skating fails and very adorable cats. Worth a follow for your morale, for sure.

@**round.boys** – really fat animals doing silly things, roundly.

@**mattzhaig, @bryonygordon, @technicallyron** – excellent authors who have written brilliantly honest books about their mental health, and continue to have the conversation on social media. Also, funny AF.

@**emotionalclub** – a controversial one due to the amount of genuinely awful brands sensationalizing mental health these days, and turning anxiety into a trend. However, I think this one is genuinely funny and makes me laugh at how shit I feel, while reminding me that I'm really not the only one who feels like this.

@**celestebarber** – rips the absolute shit out of celebrity adverts, magazine covers and bougie Instagram-model videos. Dare you not to snort.

@quarterlifepoetry – takes the piss out of how we all pretend to be perfect but really are falling apart. Relatable.

@itslennie – an emotional support blob that's always nice to receive in the DMs.

@adailycloud – even in the depths of darkness I promise at least one of these images will make you smile.

Or if they don't tickle yer pickle, how about applying these rules to accounts and only having them appear in your feed if they meet at least three of the following criteria:

- They are not showing off a traditionally 'aspirational body' and making you and yours feel crap in comparison.
- Their captions and posts are funny. One in the past six has made you chuckle out loud or want to share it with a pal.
- There is something cute to look at that makes you feel soothed.
- There is something hot to look at that makes you feel horny.
- There is something tasty to look at that makes you feel hungry (can also apply to above tbh).
- If not funny, the posts are positive and not emotionally draining/ making you feel like you should be doing more with yourself.

A friend was diagnosed with breast cancer when she was twenty-six (what the fuck?) and found that social media was actually a refreshing escape for her from the daily You-Have-Cancer onslaught. Social media – Twitter in particular, which is largely known for being a colossal mass of gits – was a space where she could be herself, and not a patient.

Social media allows us to join a community we wish we could be physically part of when we can't; you could join in with #loveisland tweets from a hospital bed, talk about the most recent political misstep when breastfeeding a child at 4 a.m., and see how many people agree with your thoughts on the new Lady Gaga album while you're waiting for a spreadsheet to download. It can allow you to be the vivacious, engaged member of society you long to be when you're unable to join likeminded people offline.

My pal Lisa told me that she loves being on Instagram these days as it's somewhere she can still be connected to the fashion and beauty worlds, and not be a mum covered in baby sick at 3 a.m. When she's breastfeeding or burping or bunjeeing and bunnyhopping (I don't know what you do with babies), she can scroll through the accounts she follows and see what's hot, and still feel connected to the world outside of nappies.

The internet is a great tool for feeling less alone when you are, in fact, physically quite the Billy-no-mates.

A simple way of feeling more 'connected' can be to simply be kind to people you already know or follow online. Telling someone that you like their house/shoes/pet cat is a simple comment that will be hugely appreciated (you are the Lord of Providing That Dopamine Hit to Someone Else), and it's a small but effective way to start to 'put yourself out there' a bit.

Even asking someone where they are to enjoy such a lovely view they've posted, congratulating someone on an achievement they're being seemingly smug about (but hey, they could be dying inside just like you! Cool!) or tagging someone in a meme that made you think of them (the modern holy grail of friendship) is a good start. Honestly, when I started a new job and, a few weeks later, a colleague DM'd me a meme… I did a little fist pump to myself. Being meme-worthy is an honour not to be taken lightly.

An internet friend is still a friend.

Social media can also be a fascinating space in which to learn new things and – gasp – improve your mind for the better. The most followed Instagram account that isn't Selena Gomez (at the time of writing) is *National Geographic* and all its associated accounts, and for good reason. We're all suckers for gorgeous nature, and we all feel awful about our plastic use. Guess what – all the cinematographers, photographers and researchers are on social media and they chuck out a shit-ton of beautiful imagery alongside informative news and ways to amp up your activism.

This is true of almost any other cause that you feel passionately about. We can all get learning – or at least follow these accounts so we feel clever when they come up in our feeds, amiright?

You're nobody 'til somebody likes you

Our brains release dopamine when we have a pleasurable experience; say, having a shag, a pint of red wine or a very garlicky bowl of mac 'n' cheese. Because it's now Instagram's world and we just have to live in it, our brains *also* release dopamine when we see that we've got a 'like'. Yup, that little red heart *controls a chemical in our brain* because of the unpredictability of the platform. If it was guaranteed that every time you put a photo onto Instagram you'd get 20,000 likes, the guessing and the chase wouldn't be there, and our brains would get pretty bored straight away.

We never know how well a post will go down, so when something's a big hit with our meagre followers and our mum, it's also a big hit for our neurotransmitters. How tragic is that? Some people (and these are 100 per cent the types of people who have a 'live life love laugh Linda' sign in their bathroom, just F your I) even *round up their most liked posts of the year*, and then *post them all in a collage as a separate post* in December to get even more bloody likes. It's all a bit *Black Mirror*, isn't it?

To receive the lusted-after double-tap and rack up the amount of self-validating 'likes' on our posts, we'd better make sure our photos look as bangin' as possible, right? And so begins the Fake Lives of Social Media, wherein everyone presents a version of their life with more than just a Valencia filter on it.

It's human nature to want to be liked and accepted. Psychotherapist Peter Klein (who specializes in treating stress, worry, anxiety, psychosis, depression and OCD – so knows what he's on about), told me that 'most validation from social media is a very direct form of feedback, as many users express their likes and dislikes more freely [online] than in person. The resulting increased sense of wellbeing can act as a positive reinforcer that some users over-rely upon.' So basically, if we got a few likes on a post once and it made us feel like we were the Queen of the internet, we'll go back and try to fish for more likes. We're gross.

'When this occurs, users run the risk of their self-esteem becoming conditional,' says Peter, 'meaning that their sense of self-worth is connected too much with how well they do something. The ease as to which validation can occur over social media increases the temptation to follow such a path.'

This makes sense; if you put a picture up on Instagram and got some 'likes' and a few cheery comments and it made you feel good about yourself, then of course you're likely to do it again and try to get the same feeling. But similarly, if you scroll through Instagram and feel depleted by the accounts that you follow and start to compare yourself and feel your self-esteem plummet – why do you keep going back? It's the FOMO (Fear of Missing Out).

I try to channel JOMO (Joy of Missing Out) by remembering that most events are actually super-tiring and someone's there who's really annoying and whoever took that photo for Instagram probably took about twenty-four before they got one they were happy with. Often, we can be having a fine time doing whatever we've chosen to be doing, but a glance at Instagram can suddenly make us feel excluded from seemingly more interesting events happening in restaurants or flats or parks we weren't invited to. When you click to open Instagram, you're actively looking at what everyone else is up to without you. I try to catch myself now, and ask myself, 'Why do I care what old school acquaintances are up to when I'm perfectly fine not knowing and continuing to eat chips in the bath?' – or whatever it may be.

Instagram is really an endless stream of adverts, promos and other people's lives that we look at while nothing is happening in our own lives (or sometimes even when something is happening and we're just too obsessed not to check Instagram when we pop to the loo).

While we have hundreds of 'friends', seeing them all post stories of themselves having a lovely time in a bougie bar on a Friday night while you're eating a wheel of cheese in an old Slipknot hoodie doesn't exactly make you feel like the social butterfly you anticipated yourself blossoming into.

Our focus has shifted to needing validation from 'likes' online rather than seeking the validation of a hug from a mate when you meet up in real actual life. It certainly makes sense for me: having access to everyone you know in the palm of your hand and being part of thirty-plus WhatsApp groups can make you feel like you're always in touch with everyone. Instagram can make you think that everyone's busy anyway, so why should you bother trying to make plans with someone when they're probably already out with more interesting and photogenic people. I get it.

JOMO is more about appreciating what you've got going on in the moment, and not surrendering to comparing it to what everyone else you know is doing.

It's a bit like mindfulness, just with a snazzier acronym.

Also, if there are people you follow who are constantly posting smug 'oh look at all the fun I'm having' posts and making you feel a bit crap, mute! Mute without restraint. Only keep those in your feed who genuinely bring you joy, and timelines will soon turn into a much calmer space.

You're so vain, you probably think this post is about you

Of course, one of the biggest gripes about Instagram is quite rightly that it's a navel-gazing vanity exercise that serves to make us all feel shit about ourselves as we scroll through reams of immaculately sculpted bodies, flawless make-up, and endless rows of abs. As mentioned… JUST STOP FOLLOWING THESE PEOPLE FOR FUCK'S SAKE.

But yeah, all right, I get it that you may not follow 'influencers' per se, but you do follow your mates, and anyone can get their hands on a few filters and a download of Facetune these days.

Of course there are people who just post selfies because they like the look of themselves, and that's absolutely fine – you do you – but then that can lead to narcissistic binges when you find yourself scrolling through your *own* social media feed and reading your *own* captions back to yourself like they're a Michelle Obama speech. Not so cool.

There's also the hardly altruistic desire we all seem to have to rub everyone's faces in it when we're having a bloody lovely time, which not only contributes to the Fake Lives of Instagram, but arguably also detracts from said lovely time because you're on your sodding phone, love.

So why do we feel the need to post these pictures of ourselves, when we're all aware of how the posts might make someone else feel? I asked some selfie fans:

- 'I look better in pictures than I do in real life and I feel like I need to share that with the world sometimes.'
- 'I do like the ego boost when I get a certain number of likes or comments, and once I've posted a selfie I am constantly checking to see how many I have.'
- 'Because I use selfies to capture moments with my family, I feel happy and reminiscent when I look back at them. I've noticed that with time I often look back and think I look better than I considered myself to look at the time I took the picture.'
- 'I actually hate looking back at my selfies once they're up. I try not to look at them too much because I pick holes in them, it's really not a great mood to start sliding on.'
- 'I don't upload many selfies, only for profile pics mainly. Recently changed my profile on Facebook and was delighted when I got over 100 likes! But at the same time I know it's not important.'
- 'I spend hours taking photos and editing the best ones before uploading a selfie. Then follows hours of validation through

likes, messages and people interacting with my selfie. It's an endorphin rush.'

- 'I need attention and it gives me a vague sensation of having an impact on people, even if it's just for a little bit.'
- 'I post selfies when I feel cute and then feel SO great seeing the likes come in, like everyone else thinks I'm cute, too. Then I feel a bit embarrassed later and like I should delete them... but I don't.'

The simple answer here is obviously to stop posting pictures of yourself, and instead post pictures of people, things, places or moments that have made you happy. Then when you're scrolling back through and laughing at your own jokes from three years ago, your brain will get a slow and steady dopamine release, rather than start questioning why you thought you were fat in that year and jeeez if you from 2013 could only see yourself now they'd be aghast. AGHAST.

When we see photos of people we love, our Brain Overlords release dopamine and oxytocin simultaneously; these are the same feel-good chemicals that thrust themselves out to us when we look at pictures of cute animals (or babies, for some people, but personally they make me do a little shudder and a sick), or when we fall in love.

Oxytocin is often referred to as 'the cuddle hormone' because our brains spurt it out when we have a squishy hug, but having oxytocin naturally in your system is way more beneficial than ten warm embraces a day. It's also released when we orgasm (and, in women, when we have our nipples stimulated), which is as good an argument for regular masturbation as I've ever heard.

If you naturally produce oxytocin from situations you find

pleasurable, you'll have increased levels of empathy – and hoooooooey does the world need more of that right now. Oxytocin also reduces your levels of stress and aggression, while upping your moral and pro-social behaviour. For anyone who's spent more than a whole day lying down in a dark room, endlessly sobbing and gasping for breath while being terrified of the outside, I'd say this one's for you.

If we can trick our brains into releasing more of these chemicals simply by looking at happy, cute stuff more (or masturbating), let's chalk that up to a win.

IN FUCKING FACT, a 2012 study showed that looking at cute images increases our attention to detail, after candidates in the study gawped at some cute baby animals for a while and then had to undertake tasks that required care and precision.[22] Compared to the candidates who didn't absorb the cuteness, they rocked it. So there, sack off the celebrity influencer twats and bring on the puppies.

You'd better work, bitch

But what about when getting likes and shares and retweets and pins is actually a part of your job? The internet has taken over the world in such an insidious, sprawling way now that half of us are doing jobs we never knew existed when we were twenty-one, let alone when we were seven and trying to say, 'When I grow up I really want to be a digital content strategist and social media lead, Mummy.'

When I worked at *Cosmopolitan* and teen website Sugarscape, a lot of my job was about getting The World to click the 'like' button on content across every digital platform available, as well as getting as many people as possible to click on articles that were being pushed out on a minute-by-minute basis.

When you work online and your job is literally judged by how many people like what you've chosen to put out to the world and the particular way you've phrased a tagline and the certain image you've selected to go with it, then you have a very tangible and instantly accessible number attached to your output. At any moment of the day you can see if people are responding well to what you're doing, and it's easy to fall into a trap of this directly relating to your mood.

If the website had slow traffic but we'd all worked really hard to produce some great-quality articles, then that was a shit mood for the rest of the day. If the hilarious Instagram post on the *Cosmopolitan* account didn't get as many likes as anticipated, then that was a shit mood for the rest of the day. If a quality piece of content that someone worked really hard on is doing well and getting lots of traffic, then HEY, let's celebrate!

This all equates to you essentially having a sordid affair with Google Analytics, which you'll look longingly at more than you will your boyfriend.

It's only natural to be emotionally invested in any piece of work that you create. YOU created it, after all. You, with the sixty-seven likes on your latest Instagram picture and a Pinterest board full of holidays you'll never be able to afford unless enough people retweet the post you've just put out on your company account. It's shamefully difficult not to be navel-gazing and self-involved when you can literally see, in real time, the number of people who are reading your work and how they are responding to it. You can even see the point in the page at which they stopped reading, for fuck's sake. Working online, as so many of us do, has deep-rooted correlations to our moods and mental health.

When I was running *Cosmo* online I found that my mood was directly related to traffic. It affected me outside of the office, too, and I'm not the only one.

Ellen works online for a national newspaper and entirely echoes my digital pain:

Traffic to my work has a huge impact on my mental health, mostly because I tie a lot of my self-worth to the work I do. I used to obsess over numbers – if I wasn't meeting targets I'd set I'd feel like a failure in all areas, not just work. I was constantly worried about getting fired and would use stats as back-up for that belief. Any negative tweets I received (and there were times I got a LOT thanks to opinion pieces about periods and sex and mental health) would add to that. I was convinced that my bosses would see that people hated me and decide they hated me too.

I used to go on live analytics on my day off and if none of my content was in the top twenty articles I would become obsessive. I'd check every half an hour and feel a need to message the people on desk to ask what was happening. I was always worrying that if things didn't go well on my days off I'd get the blame. I felt like I was doing a bad thing by taking two days off a week – which definitely isn't healthy.

But, duh, the world is online now, and if you're gonna take this all so *emotionally*, you fucking *snowflake millennial*, then where are you gonna work? Huh? It's not as if jobs are being flung about willy-nilly, is it?

Nah mate, don't quit your job – the economy is crumbling faster than a soggy rich tea biscuit and we need to take what we can get. I realize this advice is a bit rich coming from me, a woman (roar, etc.) who got so burnt out by their internet job they sacked it off to go live in the abroads alone for a few months (but that's a whole different chapter). I won't ever regret doing that, but there are things you can do to try not to get so personally attached to the numbers, which I wish I'd known at the time.

I spoke to Helen Campbell about this, as she's a career coach for creative people so comes up against this whole shebang all the time. She told me:

> *As humans, we're programmed to seek out confirmation that we exist in the world, craving attention and recognition to such an extent that even negative attention can feel better than none at all. Social media taps into that need. The 'freely' available 24/7 platforms can help us to confirm our existence and our 'worthiness'.*

When I've been looking after social media accounts in the past, I've always (shamefully) enjoyed reading through the responses to the brand's posts, because it was as if hundreds of people were having a conversation with ME, and not the brand. What a wet flannel I was.

But then, as Ellen mentioned before, it becomes addictive. Because you get so many more responses via a brand than you would on your own personal social media, there's always something new to look at if you just refresh the feed.

Helen told me that relying on any kind of work for happiness is risky and creates more unhelpful needs for validation. To have a healthy relationship with social media (but honestly, I think this applies to mostly everything) Helen suggests putting boundaries in place and deciding how much time, energy or even money you want to invest in it. There are apps available now which will force you out of your social media after you've spent a certain amount of time on them, if you need help with your boundaries.

'Finding a way to nurture ourselves – whether through sport, pastimes and/or friends and family – is somewhat essential,' says Helen. 'The key is to set up that support when you are feeling positive so that it can tide you over during the tough times.'

That's an excellent point about most things to do with depression and bad mental health, actually; you have to take advantage of the times you feel less crappy to prepare for the future when you'll be crappy again. If there's even a slight lift, it's a good idea to use that time to explain to people around you what you've been going through, what you expect to happen and what you need or don't need from them. Also, it warns them in advance that you're about to be an asshole again. Helen says:

Exploring failure can also help. If you create a campaign which doesn't produce the desired outcome, this can be a chance to learn, grow and develop. Rather than burying it under the proverbial rug, explore what happened, the decisions you made and what you learned. If you would like to make any changes as a result of that learning, try to set yourself some goals around that and choose a way of rewarding yourself for making those positive changes.

It's a tricky act to balance and one that doesn't just apply to content gremlins who work on the internet. Ellen, a much wiser woman than me, seems to have a good strategy:

I'm working hard on valuing myself beyond my work – that's been a huge project in progress this year. I'm trying to focus on other things that make me happy and make me who I am. It's why I'm trying to do volunteer work at the moment so that my days off are still filled with me doing something that makes me feel worthy, but without stats to focus on.

I'm also working on valuing measures of success outside of numbers. I'm focusing on if I had a fun day, if I'm proud of what I've worked on and if I think what I'm doing could have an impact on someone. With everything I put on the internet I'm trying to ask what the purpose of it is. It needs to be doing something, whether that's changing views, raising awareness of an issue, getting policy changed, making someone feel less weird and alone (that's a big one), or just making someone feel happy for a bit.

If I'm not doing any of those things, why am I putting this out on the internet? If I am doing these things, I think they're more valuable than the number of unique visitors to an article or the number of retweets something gets.

Counsellor Peter Klein adds that if you do just *put the phone down* and try to *stop* checking the stats all the goddam time, your mental health will improve. YES, PETER WE KNOW THIS,

HOW DO WE DO IT, THOUGH? 'This is often a difficult step as those affected will frequently notice a strong urge to engage in their unhelpful behaviours. Eventually those urges lessen, and thoughts surrounding negative feedback will start fading.

'It also helps to remember that feedback will relate to the company and not be indicative of a negative statement towards the individual that produces the content.'

Exactly. It's so easy to take things personally when you've put so much effort into it, but anything that's put out via a company is essentially *about the company* and not you personally.

WhatsApp all about, Alfie?

Not technically falling under the social media umbrella (which is idiotic because it is a medium on which we socialize… yeah, come at me, Media Studies GCSE terminology) but definitely falling prey to our collective addictive and narcissistic tendencies is dear ol' blue-tick churning, anxiety-inducing WhatsApp.

At this point, it's fairly widely known that flitting between four or five 'messaging/interaction-based' apps feeds wildly into our natural impatience for instant gratification, validation and information. This, what a surprise, gives us light anxiety and ye olde FOMO. Now that we've got WhatsApp in our hands, it's literally like we're walking around with a souped-up version of MSN Messenger in our pockets, and I think we all remember how big a part that dial-up modem and Blink-182-lyrics-as-a-screen-name played in our formative years.

You've probably got people in your WhatsApp inbox that have turned off the blue ticks because, like, they're so, like, *above* all that, and they're super-carefree and don't need people to know when they're gonna reply or if they've seen their message or not. They're so breezy and chilled and nonchalant and bohemian about it all they're probably running barefoot through a hemp field right now and listening to 'Orinoco Flow'.

Bull. Shit.

OK, so maybe these people are carefree *now*, but I would pretty much guarantee that the reason they obliterated the blue ticks from their lives in the first place was because they were becoming a bit too Icarus-into-the-sun with it all. Getting rid of the blue ticks helps. Do it right now, and while you're there get rid of the 'last seen online' thing, too (then please come back to the book, I have separation anxiety).

I saw someone tweet once that it should cost everyone a fiver to set up and join a new WhatsApp group, and I couldn't agree more. I've had WhatsApp groups set up for going to the CINEMA, for fuck's sake. For going to the PARK, and for *getting the same train together one time ever*. They serve a dual purpose (both shite, if you hadn't seen that coming already) of allowing us to spend hours of our days talking absolute bollocks with five groups of similar people, and also to feel like a worthless, friendless tumbleweed when you look at your phone and don't have any notifications, or you've been left on read.

OK, so there are three options here (and there's nothing stopping you doing them all if you're a super-keeno):

1. **Leave your groups.** Yeah, this could make you seem like a stone-cold bitch, but fuck it. Leave them. 90 per cent of group chats are full of mindless guff anyway, and the lack of notifications building up while you're at work is honestly a very soothing experience. People who you want to speak

to will get in touch with you. The rest of the stuff, you'll miss out on and be glad of it.

2. **Turn off WhatsApp.** Leave your phone on 3G (don't connect it to Wi-Fi) and go to your WhatsApp settings and turn off WhatsApp use for mobile data. This is likely the biggest use of your internet anyway so don't come crying to me about bills. Then, when you're ready to read any messages/send any yourself, you can either turn it back on or connect to Wi-Fi, and have a little WhatsApp sesh on your own terms rather than it pellet-gunning into your life throughout the day while you're just trying to use Google Maps.

3. **Airplane mode.** Just fuck it and turn it all off but still be able to see what time it is.

The clapbacks

So, what could you say if some mate who fancies themselves an amateur psychologist suggests that you 'just stay off Instagram for a bit, hun'? Perhaps:

'Thanks! But actually I'm using social media to only look at things that make me feel good and it's really helping – so I've muted you, soz.'

'Actually, I've found that connecting to a community of like-minded people who have the same struggles as me is really useful – so I've muted you, soz.'

We can use social media for a positive effect if we're not total dicks about it. If you're feeling overwhelmed by every status update you read and news push notification that you get, just turn them the fuck off. *Everything* is competing for space in your brain, and I for one don't want to forget the words to anything by Celine Dion because I've had too many WhatsApp group messages. It's about being aware of what you're consuming and questioning how people you follow and the content they produce makes you feel. You feel shit enough already, so if something doesn't make you actively happier or more amused, sack it off.

CHAPTER 6

Your boyfriend is so fit though, babe

Having a gorgeous and loving partner is incredible, sure, but hiding a mental illness from them will exhaust you to your unexercised core.

Why would you want to show them that you're crumbling on the inside? Why would you let your tears out in front of them when you can save the emotion for when they're out at the shops and the tears just naturally spurt out of your face like water bursting through a dam? Why would you reveal to them – the person you want never to leave you – how desperate and broken you're really feeling? You'd both have more fun if you just got your shit together and ignored it while they were around, and there's a strong chance they'll 'go off you' if they see how dark you really are.

This is the person you want to look forward to seeing you and to want to see you more, not the person you want to delay coming home because they have no idea what particular shade of misery you'll be coloured in that day.

Why would you talk to them about how miserable you are, when they've been on the receiving end of so many 'I'm sorry' WhatsApps that it's not as if they can't see it for themselves?

I'm sorry for cancelling. I'm sorry for being quiet. I'm sorry I'm not coming out. I'm sorry I've been bad company. I'm sorry for leaving early. I'm sorry I feel like I'm dying inside and I'm too scared to talk about it with you because you'll start worrying and I don't want the attention, and you'll want to leave me if I show you how I'm really feeling and stop putting on this front, and you'll feel like you can't leave me because it would be cruel to leave someone with a mental health problem, so you'll just find someone else anyway and feel guilty about it and then you'll hate yourself and resent me and the whole thing will be easier if I just say I'm not feeling well and go to bed. P.S. Also can you pick up some bog roll and a Twix xoxo.

Telling the whole truth

When I was in a really bad way, I never talked to my ex-boyfriend properly about how staggeringly awful I felt. I never let him see me cry properly, and I never opened up fully about the extent of the illness, and how I sometimes just sat in the dark for hours and hours with hot, silent tears streaming down my face, and my belly feeling hollow and electrified.

I never told him about crying at work, on the way to work, on the way home from work, and sometimes when I went to the bathroom in the middle of a film we were watching at home because I couldn't hold it in any longer (the tears, but the pee, too, I guess). It's not as if I didn't love him and trust him implicitly, it was the fear of watching his face change as he realized I'd gone absolutely and completely mad. As he realized I was deranged and unlovable, and he panicked about just who the fuck he'd spent the past sixteen years of his life with. It's the pressure of asking someone else to be aware of you and how you're feeling, when you don't know how to manage how you're feeling yourself.

It's the awareness of a huge, ugly, wet, crying burden that you're putting onto their shoulders. It's the worry that they'll tip-toe around you and be overly fake happy to make sure you're not going to off yourself. It's not wanting to worry them. It's not wanting to be immediately shipped off to some island where you're made to wear straitjackets and be spoon-fed gruel and sing a prescribed daily chorus of 'All Things Bright and Beautiful'. It's the dreaded 'So, how are you *feeling*?' with the associated head-tilt that comes from anyone you've dared ever mention it to in the past.

It's everything.

So let's just carry on and pretend.

Let's pretend when we're in bed, lying next to each other in the darkness and you're falling asleep. Let's pretend that I'm not forcing myself to lie stone-still so that you don't notice the shaking from the crying. Let's pretend that I slept 'yeah, good, thanks' instead of waking up at 4 a.m. like clockwork, gasping for breath as a scorching poker of pain stabbed me in the chest, and feeling myself sinking as the sadness spreads and spirals through me like dark ink leaking onto a page. Let's pretend the hotel has 'quite lumpy beds actually' and the mascara smudged all over the pillow is 'ugh, typically crap make-up remover'. Let's just keep pretending.

Well, this is cheerful, isn't it? Anyone know any jokes?

I first told my then-partner – let's call him Dré (because that's his name) – that I was depressed one evening when we were in bed, about to go to sleep. It was a weeknight, we had work in the morning and we'd both been tired and sensible that evening, and watched a few episodes of *Black Mirror* or something before heading to bed. Lights off. Hiding in the shadows. Dré was probably just drifting off into sleep when I interrupted his peace, simply by saying, 'I got a new prescription from the doctor today.'

'Oh? What for? I didn't realize you were sick.'

'Antidepressants.'

'… I had no idea you felt like that.'

'Yeah. But it's fine.'

I mean, it wasn't fucking fine, was it? It was shite, and the feeling of misery had built up to such an intense pressure it was all I could do to believe I wasn't actually walking around wearing a big SAD GALS CLUB sandwich board over my clothes. I thought it must have been *so* obvious, *so* painted on my face. In reality, all that was painted on there was the pretence, while the paint cans were exploding inside.

When one person's depressed, at least two people will suffer with it. Hell, sometimes ten, as it seeps out of you and into all your relationships, whether personal or professional. Such a thrill.

Anyway, at that point I was on the third round of antidepressants, and felt like I had to tell Dré because the last two trial runs had made me a bit loopy, which, teamed with the charming hypochondriac tendencies I had developed at that time, basically ignited a will to tell him simply so he would know the cause of my fainting if I suddenly passed out in the bathroom or something.

If you have a partner from whom you're keeping your struggles, please try not to feel guilty or ashamed. I hid my mental health problems from Dré for years, sugaring over the top of the darkness to make the illness more palatable for him, and so do heaps of other people just like you and me. I'm not saying you should keep it a secret forever because I really do encourage you to tell your partner about what's happening to you, but don't rush into it. Everything's on your terms.

Back when Dré and I were still together I interviewed him about my depression for this book, which was odd and sad and felt a bit like we were doing some kind of very unsexy role play, but was also pretty enlightening and made me realize I should have asked him these questions years ago instead of tip-toeing around the subject and not wanting to upset him/put him off me/make him worry.

It's so easy to get caught up in thoughts of what you *assume* people think of you, but as the saying goes: **thoughts are not facts. You'll never know until you ask.** I would urge you to ask these questions of your partner, housemate or whoever you're closest to. There's no point me dressing it up like a glossy magazine interview ('Dré was languishing across an old sofa in North London, his dark, chocolatey eyes looking pensive and wise,' etc.), so I'll just write out some of the transcript for you here, you lucky thing.

> K: *So, this will be a laugh. [Laughs nervously.] Do you remember when I first told you I was depressed?*
> D: *I do. I remember the first time you told me, but it was kind of like… it was a bit more of a gradual thing for me to understand. I didn't really understand that you were actually, like, fully depressed, it was more… I thought you were saying that you were feeling a bit depressed. Not like you were Suffering With Depression, just that you were feeling down.*
> K: *What do you remember about that conversation?*
> D: *I remember you not looking at me. I remember not really*

fully comprehending what you meant. I remember you saying when you were first going onto medication.

K: Ah. That was actually the third time I was trying medicine but I didn't tell you before that.

D: Woah. How long had you been on medication before that then?

K: I'd tried a few different ones short term but they hadn't worked out, and I didn't want to tell you because I was embarrassed.

D: Oh, right.

K: Do you remember how you felt when I told you?

D: Not really. I don't remember having a reaction to it. You played it down anyway. It was something that I just acknowledged and thought it was something that we would work through. I didn't have a strong reaction to it.

K: Was it a surprise?

D: Yeah, it was. But probably me not having a strong reaction to it was a bit of denial that it would be a long-term thing, and me being in a little bit of shock – not like, need-a-cup-of-tea shock. I hadn't seen it coming. It did make sense when you said it, though.

K: How differently did you think of me when I said it?

D: I didn't think of you differently.

K: Did you feel like you had to behave differently around me?

D: Ah. Well, I mean, that's an interesting question really because yes and no. I didn't feel like I needed to tip-toe around you or anything, but you are saying that there's something wrong with you so I am gonna have to... it is going to be different, in the same way that if you said you had any kind of illness, there's gonna be an impact.

K: *Different how?*

D: *Well, being more understanding of the fact that you're not being moody, you're depressed. If you've gone for a lie down, it's not because you're in a mood with me or because you're annoyed at me or I've done something to piss you off, it's because you're depressed.*

K: *Oh. I never thought you'd think of it like that.*

D: *Why? What did you think?*

K: *I just thought you'd think I was shit and boring and always going to lie down and be on my own, and would have just thought that I was a crap girlfriend and you'd want a new one.*

D: *Well, I didn't.*

Oh, Alanis Morissette would have a field day with that one, wouldn't she? While I worried about being a crap girlfriend through sharing my mental health struggles, I would actually have been a crapper girlfriend if I'd kept it all to myself. Dré even said that 'it made sense' when I told him I was depressed, after previously thinking that there was seemingly no reason for me needing to be alone or silent for a while and that I was avoiding him, or was just being a moody cow. Oops.

Personally, I'm not sure how glad I am that I told Dré, which is probably not what I'm supposed to say here, but I'm being honest. I mean, it's all in a fucking book now so he'd have found out at some point, but it did feel like exposing my biggest secret and that he (and anyone else who knew) would think I was being overdramatic, hearkening back to my emo days of 2003, and that I should just get a grip.

I later found out that my example of telling Dré super-casually is essentially textbook depressive. Oh good.

'Talking about depression can be emotionally challenging, which can motivate people to be really brief when opening up or try to underplay their difficulties,' Peter Klein told me – so if you too told your partner in a very blasé fashion, you're not being a dick, you're just being depressed. 'Both tendencies are common hallmarks of depression,' he confirmed. 'It's important to try and be as open as possible and honest as possible, while not downplaying the concern.'

After I had told Dré, I still didn't really let my guard down around him and show him how miserable I was. I'd disappear upstairs to 'lie down' in the dark for a few hours or cancel group plans to go home alone instead. That's about the extent of how much (I thought) I let him see, because how miserable is it to live with a sack of sad shit? How exhausting? It's not his fault my brain has broken, and – despite knowing that the stigma needs to change and that I'm not alone in feeling this way – I'm still deeply embarrassed to talk about my mental health with people I care about. I do cry in public a lot though, to get it out before I get home (hi, end carriage on the 18.42 train to Alexandra Palace), and find it's a lot easier to write about it in a Word document than it is to say out loud.

Talking to Dré about it for said Word document was really difficult, but it felt meaningful.

K: *What is helpful for me to tell you about how I'm feeling? Or what's unhelpful?*
D: *I can't think of anything that would be unhelpful. It's important that you say how you're feeling, and if you're feeling like you want to be alone then you need to say. Go lie in the dark room. I do think you need to say more sometimes, rather than trying to hide it.*

K: But if I didn't try to hide it then I'd never leave the dark room.

I spoke to a gal called Mel about her struggles to tell her ex-partner about her depression, and she agreed that 'sometimes writing down how you feel can help, as it can be hard to express such deep, painful and frightening emotions verbally. Those who haven't experienced mental illness (lucky them) cannot have any conception of how crippling it is; how hard it is to get up in the morning, cope with normal social interactions and just function.'

Referring to depression as a third person can help both you and someone else understand that it's an illness. It's not part of you and it's really not how you're *choosing* to behave. It's latched itself onto you and you don't want to let it in. People call it the black dog. People call it the dark cloud. People call it Gretel. Sometimes I call it Nigel (honestly, I've never met anyone called Nigel that I liked, have you?), or refer to the depression demons and also tended to text Dré an emoji of a raincloud (because I'm emo and dramatic) when I was feeling terrible and was cancelling on plans. But does this feel like an easy excuse? Just chucking over a raincloud text and then nobody can be mad at you for bailing, and your friend/partner/gentleman lover is the one left having to make excuses to everyone?

K: What about when I send you the raincloud emoji text? How does that work for ya?

D: I find that it's a good way of communicating it actually. It says how you're feeling without having to write it. I interpret that as you needing space and you're feeling worse than usual. Is that what it means?

K: *Yeah, that I'm feeling really horrible and down, and am probably mid-cry and just need to be alone in the dark. Does it feel like a cop-out when I send it?*

D: *Nope.*

K: *How much have you had to make excuses for me when I've rainclouded or cancelled at the last minute?*

D: *I just say that you're not very well. It's not an excuse, it's the truth, and nobody ever asks what specifically is wrong.*

K: *How much do you feel like you get the shit version of me and my friends get the good version?*

D: *Um… I don't feel like I get the shit version. I wouldn't say that you're a completely different person. If there was someone on the sofa next to us now and then as soon as they left you'd morph into a different person, that'd be different. At home we can still laugh and have a good time, and you can still be grumpy when we're out. You're obviously gonna be more inclined to go have a lie-down or be quiet or… you're more inclined to express your depression when you're home because it's a comfortable environment and you can't keep it bottled up all the time. You can't lie down on the floor of the Tube or in a pub, so it's going to be when you're at home.*

It's exhausting, being fake happy. It takes up all my energy, and then I end up going to bed early anyway because I'm so knackered from wading through treacle and keeping up a chirpy facade.

I do realize how lucky I am that I could keep up a pretence at all, and am fully aware that there are others (which at one point was me) who are completely unable to perform a happy charade because their mental health is in a much graver state of turmoil.

I realize this. I've been like this. I'm not like this anymore, which is why I've got enough distance to wang on about it in a book. I hope you're not like this. If you are, you're not the only one. I promise.

But what if your partner ends up being a total dick about it?

Peter also told me that through his counselling he of course sees many different people in all kinds of different relationship dynamics. It's true, some people go out with right fuckwits. So what happens then? Peter says:

> *The first step is to ensure that the right dynamic exists in order to learn that opening up is a positive experience. When opening up, a good first step is to describe how the depression is experienced. Depression will affect many people differently and the expressions of depression one experiences need to be understood in order to best describe it to someone else. If someone does not yet have that insight, then it can be helpful to talk about their depression in a way that they can make sense of it.*

So, while it's fine to say, 'I'm depressed and I feel awful all the time,' it's not actually very helpful. A clearer way of expressing it would be to say, 'I'm depressed and I feel absolutely exhausted all the time. I have really little energy and often need to lie down in the dark, and sometimes cry. I'm not avoiding you, I just really need the rest and the alone time.'

Of course, there will be ignorant people who won't try to

understand what you're going through, despite your being as explanatory and informative as that dictionary woman off of *Countdown*. If someone's not giving you the support you need after you've explicitly illustrated exactly what would make your life more bearable, they're not worth keeping around.

Unsurprisingly, this is a common occurrence at The Sad Gals Club.

While I was writing this, I spoke to a fellow sad gal called Keira. Keira had to break up with her ex-boyfriend after he was entirely unsupportive of her mental health struggles, and responded in a way that's undoubtedly common, and perhaps understandable if you're a total fucking imbecile: he was supportive at first and helped her look into treatment and counselling, but then got cranky and impatient when Keira's mental health wasn't immediately 'fixed'.

His support eventually gave way to impatience, ignorance, and a total lack of empathy once Keira started to take steps to look after herself.

Once she began taking medication, her boyfriend couldn't understand why she wasn't getting better. Because they had effectively 'found a solution' in his mind, he couldn't understand why she was still sometimes unable to get out of bed or shower, and how she felt so low still that she needed to take time away from work.

Keira told me how his messages of support and love soon felt hollow and were replaced with emotional blackmail; he said he needed her and was feeling lonely and abandoned because she needed so much time alone. Keira eventually broke up with him because he wasn't taking her mental health seriously, and when she met someone else eighteen months later, she was understandably reluctant to talk about her mental health struggles after Mr

Fuckwad was such a damp squib to her before. She didn't want to 'ruin things' with her new partner, but it turns out he's incredibly supportive and understands that she wants a boyfriend, not a carer, but that the relationship will take compromise to work with her mental health struggles.

Let's talk about sex, baby

Being depressed certainly fucks with the fucking, doesn't it?

Depression also has a very odd effect on your libido. Personally I've found (Mum, Dad, skip this bit, please) that rather than being the proud and careful owner of a sex drive that thrums along at a steady wavelength and can be heightened or lowered depending on whether I'm having a lovely snog or reading about Republicans, it's now at the extreme ends of both options – but it has to be coaxed out.

The engine can still get started, but it takes a hell of a long time to find the damn keys.

Definitely largely due to the medication that I'm currently taking, any glimpse of libido that I previously enjoyed has had a thick, Aran wool blanket smothered over it and neatly tucked in at the edges. BUT, there are some days when, if an attractive person pays me the remotest, slightest bit of sexual attention, the blanket will catch fire and whip off and I'll be as raging as Austin Powers in a hot tub.

Why? It could actually be due to the depressed part of your brain 'lighting up' around all the sexy times, and distracting you from the painful ache that it's usually churning out. Instead of misery, you're being overtaken completely by desire, and your brain is telling you to follow that through because that Aran blanket being on fire feels alarmingly better than the usual darkness.

Although, let's be realistic, you won't find yourself being chatted up by many attractive strangers if you continue to stay lying in a dark room alone in silence. If you *do* venture out of the house, chances are you look like utter shit. I'm sorry, love, but it's true. This is fair enough, though. Getting out of the house can seem like a tragically enormous mountain to climb, and when just making it outside and on the way to work is an achievement in itself, why should you have to comb your hair or check if you're wearing a clean top?

This fact was oh-so-hilariously brought home to me one morning in the Pret a Manger on Trafalgar Square (I'm sure I'm merely one of many who've had an epiphany next to the tuna baguettes). I was trundling in one morning to get a pint of caffeine, and bumped into a member of a boyband I used to interview once, sometimes twice a week when I worked at a teen website (Sugarscape.com, now folded, but the best job ever). He held the door open for me as I shuffled inside, and actually said 'woah' when he recognized me, because I looked so rough. It was fairly humiliating. We had an awkward 'so how are you, where are you working now?' stop-n-chat, and he looked me very slowly up and down with an expression of disbelief on his face.

It's a particular low point, being given a pitying look by a man who once wore a white suit to please Louis Walsh.

'You look… um, well?' he muttered, as his eyes locked on to an enormous unidentified stain on my jumper, which I was sporting with greasy hair, an extra two stone in weight, and last night's cry-mascara probably still smudged on my face.

Mortified, on the way to the office I bought a bottle of dry shampoo, which was liberally applied in the bathroom after I'd washed my face and tried to at least lessen the mystery splotch on my jumper. It sounds like nothing, but it felt like a big realization that I'd let myself go to shit – and I needed an embarrassing encounter with a boybander to remind me of that. Tragic.

While I'm a firm believer in not giving a crap about what other people think of you, it's much easier said than done. Ultimately, I wasn't rubbing the grease out of my hair in preparation for future popstar tête-à-têtes near the porridge, but more in desperation to try to get some of myself back. For me. That's what it's about: doing things for yourself. If you put too much pressure on yourself to keep up a pretence for other people – whether it's a partner or family or a housemate you don't even like that much – you'll crumble. If you lean too heavily on the support of a loved one, at some point they're going to have to move away an inch and you're likely to (quite literally in my case) fall over.

I'm not in the Sad Gals Club but my partner is – WTF do I do?

To be in a relationship with someone who has depression must fucking suck, let's be honest. I've spoken to a lot of people who agree that as a partner of someone with depression, it can feel like their own feelings are – or should be – dwarfed in comparison to the feelings of the depressed person, and that anything they feel is insignificant compared to the horrors happening to their depressed love. So the depressed person keeps their feelings to themselves, so does the partner, and that depression slowly, insidiously erodes the relationship. Fun!

As much as the depressed party in the couple is feeling awful, it's pretty damn likely that the non-depressed partner is also feeling a tad dubious about the situation and is also trying not to fuck things up, albeit in very different ways. What if they say the wrong thing and it turns out to be upsetting or offensive? What if they're not sensitive enough? What if they're over-sensitive? What if they wake up one morning and find they're lying next to a corpse? What an absolute LOL it all must be.

Peter Klein points out that if you're told that your partner is depressed, it might feel like it's on you to 'fix' them – but, it's of course absolutely not. Your depressed amour needs support and comfort more than anything and won't be looking to you for solutions. He told me:

> *It's initially not important to come up with suggestions or solutions, but to create a welcoming and rewarding environment for the partner to open up. This will make them feel comfortable with opening up and therefore create the basis for further insight and potential improvements. Helping a partner choose the right kind of treatment can also be helpful. The numerous support services out there can make this task seem overwhelming and an often surprisingly helpful resource can be a local GP.*
>
> *It's important to remember that if a partner opens up about being depressed, this is not a negative reflection on oneself. Feelings of guilt or shame need to be understood within this context.*

That's a great point actually. I'd never thought that Dré might feel like me being glum is a bad reflection on him, and that seems like an important thing to remember when talking to anyone you love about how you feel: **it's really not anyone's fault, your brain has just caught fire and gone wonky. Depression isn't an illness that can be loved out of you.**

To get some more opinions, I spoke to a non-sad gal called Hannah, who is in a relationship with a man who suffers from debilitating depression. She told me very honestly that when he's going through a particularly bad time, it can make her feel a little needy as when he's depressed, he finds it difficult to express his love and affection. Even though Hannah understands what's happening and knows the feelings are there, it doesn't make it any easier to live with. 'I got so angry and affronted by this at first,' she told me, 'even though I understood what was happening, which ultimately made me realize just how much validation I needed from other people. While I still need more than a lot of people, I was able to work on that, and am now much more confident in myself and less reliant on others' opinions of me – an unexpected effect, but a welcome one!'

It sounds like going out with a depressive doesn't exactly do wonders for your self-esteem, so having a friend (or therapist) who can build you up is fairly essential if you want to keep the relationship going.

But then, how can you provide support to a depressed partner without becoming overbearing or ineffective? From personal experience and from asking around, the most popular response from depressed people is 'just be there and hug me while I cry'.

This sounds (to me) like the best kind of support: non-judge-mental, present, kind and silent. What I would say to a partner or close friend of someone in this kind of darkness is just to be there for them. Physically. Be next to them. Read a book next to them or do your work next to them or quietly watch a film next to them. Be physically close to them. Draw them a bath. Draw them a picture! That would actually be quite lush.

Make them some tea. Don't ask anything of them and don't try to push them into activity or cleanliness. Telling someone – even in a light-hearted way – that it's about time they get into the shower because they're starting to smell a bit ripe is not supportive. Preparing someone a relaxing bath that smells delicious and has some soothing low lighting is a much better shout, or putting on some fresh bed sheets and candles if you don't have the space for a tub.

But this is really only if the partner can cope with the depression. Depression is a lot to take on as a partner; despite not having it yourself, you have to navigate the unknown with someone you love and who you desperately want to be better. Sometimes the honest truth is that it's better for the partner to leave.

My wonderful friend Hayley was with her ex-partner for ten years. He was depressed and an alcoholic, and although she loved him dearly, eventually the right thing for her to do was to end the relationship. She told me:

He didn't really tell me that he was depressed. I had no idea he was drinking until I started having to take him to hospital. Eventually I realized the extent of the drinking and depression was unavoidable as he was living a bit of a nocturnal life. We had the curtains closed most of the time, and while I was leading a pretty normal life he was just stuck in this enormous rut.

As a partner of someone with depression I think you just feel helpless. I tried so much to help him and help him get help, but ultimately it has to be that person who does it and you can't do it for them.

The hardest thing was knowing that I had to leave, but that by doing so, he would then sink even further. But he had to do that in order to get to a properly rock-bottom place and realize he had to get proper help.

I found it extremely frustrating that I couldn't fix him, and it was hard because he hated himself so much that he couldn't understand why I would love him.

It's hard and horrible enough to end a relationship even if both of you are glowing healthy specimens in the absolute prime of your lives, let alone if one of you is severely depressed.

But don't worry, the depressed person can't feel feelings and probably won't even notice you've gone. Yippee!

OK, that was a lie.

Ending a relationship because of depression is just the same as ending a relationship because of another thing, you just have to take a bit of extra time and care with the depressed party as they're not exactly having a ball at the moment anyway. It will probably feel like kicking a puppy in the face – there's no way around that, but if it's what's best then it's more cruel to hang around and fake it.

When looking for different experiences around this, I spoke to a girl called Rebecca who told me about ending her marriage as an indirect result of her husband's depression. She told me:

My ex-husband would never admit that he was depressed, although now that I know he was, his dramatic mood swings and paranoia all make a lot more sense. At first I just thought he was being moody.

Um, hello, so did Dré. This phenomenal sample size of two must mean this is a hugely common misconception.

His moods were so unpredictable at times that it made living with him quite a challenge. Not all the time – I'd hate for you to think that he was not a kind man, or that the eighteen years we had together were miserable – as that wasn't the case. He was fun and thoughtful and occasionally romantic. But he was also very, very moody.

Sometimes he'd be in a really great mood, I'd leave the room for fifteen mins to do something and by the time I got back, his mood would have changed and he'd be quiet, sullen and uncommunicative. Sometimes it was like treading on eggshells around him – I couldn't say anything without him snapping at me. Sometimes he could barely bring himself to look at me, never mind touch me.

Towards the very end of our relationship he finally, after much persistence from me, asked the doctor for antidepressants. But by that point, our relationship was too broken for the medication to make any difference to us.

Nowadays I rarely see him, so I don't know what his life is like at the moment. I tried to support him, tried to be patient, tried to help him, to ignore the moods, to put on a brave face – for eighteen years! But then I got to the point where I'd had enough. And so that was the end of that.

How to support a partner with depression

Don't take their actions personally. They are depressed and self-involved. Needing space is not about needing a break from you, it's about needing to be alone. Give them space.

Support rather than push. Let them lean on you and let them know it's OK not to be OK. Let them cry if they need to. Let them be silent if they want to be.

Don't treat them like an ill person. As in, don't walk on eggshells for fear they might crumble. Don't not ask them questions because you're worried they've briefly forgotten they're depressed and you'll be serving them a harsh reminder; they haven't forgotten, and if they're in a seemingly better mood then it's probably the best time to talk to them.

Remember that you might need support, too. It can be knackering living with a depressed person. Don't forget your own needs and that you're absolutely entitled to feel worn out from it, too. It's not all totally about them.

How to help your partner help you, if you're depressed

Tell them what you need, they can't read your mind. Dré thought he could read my emotions from my face. He couldn't entirely. Nobody can. Communicate clearly what you need and why. 'I need to lie down because I'm feeling a bit grey' is much better than just walking off and shutting the door in silence. 'I need some alone time this evening, but let's hang out tomorrow' will be better received than 'fuck off'.

Let them know what's helped you before – if anything. Again, it's helpful to talk about this during the windows of time when you're not feeling Peak Gloom. It's worth saying, 'Hey, I know I can disappear into the darkness sometimes – I can't control it, but sometimes it helps if I am on my own for the evening/am distracted by loud and glittering theatre productions/have a bath/ go for a walk – but I won't want to so you'll have to force me and pretend we're doing it because YOU really want to go for a walk.'

Provide them with some information about depression – whether it's a website, this book or just you talking it through in your own words, explaining that depression is an illness, not a bad mood. Depression produces uncontrollable side effects and your partner really should not take it personally if you need to be alone or if you seem sad or irritated. Remind them that although it might seem like you hate them sometimes, you really don't; it's just what happens when the gas on your brain-fire is turned up.

Eventually, my depression hugely contributed to the end of my relationship with Dré. As well as making you a ball of misery, depression has other great aspects, like making you very cranky, irritable and likely to have a go at someone for not meeting you at the right entrance of a train station instead of just giving them a loving hug because you haven't seen them for a month.

Living with someone who has depression is, I'm sure, pretty monstrous. Dré told me that he never knew 'which version' of me he would be coming home to. Would I be cracking open the wine, singing in the kitchen and putting on a happy face while I drank, drank and drank, and then kept on drinking when he went to bed? Would I already be in bed, in the dark, crying? Would I be a seething mass of rage and snap at him for everything? Or would I be trying to act normal but not doing a very good job at trying to tell a super-fun story from work while I was crying? What an absolute extravaganza of fun.

I loved Dré too much to show him myself without the filter on, really. I didn't want him to see how utterly miserable I really was as I didn't want him to worry or to blame himself – even the scenarios that I mentioned before had a layer of pretence about them so I wouldn't show my true misery. I think that's why depression manifests in anger so much, because there's not another way to channel out your toxic feelings. But, by hiding and pretending and putting on a front to try to keep him close, I ended up pushing him away.

I don't have the answers to the questions about how the fuck to love someone when you're depressed and want to die. I know that talking about wanting to die isn't great for your partner to hear – and that it's difficult for someone on the outside to understand the difference between wanting to die to stop the pain and actively thinking about ending your life, but I also know that not talking about it adds to the pressure cooker of doom inside you.

The problem with most dysfunctional relationships – whether it be romantic, office-based, or with your siblings or friends – is that the communication is buggered. With depression and all its hilarious complexities and contradictions, I really have no idea if being more open about it would have helped my relationship. Neither does Dré.

Dré was an incredible partner and we loved each other ferociously. We still do and I don't think I have the capacity to ever love anyone as much as I love Dré, but depression in a relationship will affect you both, and it wasn't fair for me to keep him locked in my prison cell.

Having a wonderful, gorgeous boyfriend doesn't really do much to make your depression go away. Losing that wonderful, gorgeous boyfriend doesn't help either.

Now I just want to be alone. Which is bad news for all of those boybanders…

The clapbacks

So, what to say when some first-class div asks you how you can possibly be depressed when you've got such a lovely boyfriend/girlfriend/spouse/illicit lover?

'Yes, I do, and of course it's hard for them too, but they're being really supportive, thanks.'

'Unfortunately being depressed has sod all to do with how fit my boyfriend is and everything to do with being a mental illness, but he really is hot, right? Let's talk about that.'

'Oh WAIT, yes! I'll just get him to fuck me back to happiness. Cheers.'

Ultimately, it's going to be very difficult to get better if you keep your illness a secret. You wouldn't try to hide a broken foot from your partner, and hobble around on it every day with a fake grimace plastered on, pretending you can't feel the crushing pain and just silently hoping that it'll heal itself. It won't. Neither will this. Depression is an illness, and ill people need support and help. If you're struggling to find a way to tell your partner – hell, why not show them this chapter? It's designed to help them as well as you. You are not the first or last person to go through this. Telling your partner won't be a magical cure, but explaining your illness might very well dilute the pain.

CHAPTER 7

Why don't you try making some new friends, darlin'?

Loneliness is something we tend to associate with adverts showing the elderly cooped up in their house with the heating off, desperate for a knock from a neighbour or a phone call from a relative with only their slowly dying dog for company.

Loneliness, visually, seems to be someone sad and alone at a party, not dancing with anyone. Or when the 102-year-old in front of you in a supermarket queue is buying dog food and two cans of John Smith's, which makes you want to hug him and go round for a cuppa.

Studies have shown that it is, in fact, us groovy millennials who are the loneliest generation to ever exist (well, since surveys began, cave people weren't exactly being asked to rate their loneliness out of ten for YouGov).[23, 24]

Of course, being lonely may very well lead to feelings of depression, and being depressed makes it gargantuously more difficult to socialize. What a joyful vicious circle of doom.

It's great to be able to stay connected online and with messaging in our phones and TVs, and probably kettles soon enough, but we need hugs.

My loneliness is killing me

Being alone is not the same as being lonely. We all have different needs: some need connection every day, some are satisfied with a few deep connections every month. People need different levels of social intimacy, and can feel lonely when surrounded by others, too. Loneliness is painful, and our bodies developed pain sensations to alert us to problems so that we can fix things. If you ignore the pain of loneliness it can become chronic.

Loneliness is officially identifying the gap between the amount of friends or company that you have versus the amount that you'd actually really like to have. Some people have no friends and love it, some people have no friends and hate it desperately – and kooky American sitcoms about bunches of LOLsome millennial pals who all live in the same street and hang out before, during and after work every day aren't exactly doing their bit to paint a picture of reasonable normality.

Alone time is brilliant. It's natural to crave some solitude if you've spent a while surrounded by people. Being 'peopled-out' is very real, but so is being 'people-less' when you really want to be 'people-full'. If you spend a lot of time alone and really, truly would rather the peace of it and your own thoughts (however dark they may be) than spending time making chit-chat about the weather and the government and oh-have-you-SEEN-Gemma's-new-car-yet with others, then great. Fantastic. I crave alone time constantly, and often go for meals, drinks, cinema trips, weekend breaks and even months of travelling as a solo artiste. But if you yearn for mates, that'll be where loneliness strikes.

Technology, while great for using social media, dating or friend-ship apps to meet people you'd never usually encounter, it's also now a huge barrier to IRL interaction. Gone are the days when people would have a cute, accidental meeting in a coffee shop because they were sitting on the same communal table and 'just got to talking'. Now these people have laptops and headphones and essentially an enormous, electrified fence around them, brandishing a sign that says, 'Don't you even think about beginning to try to talk to me because I'm actually very busy and important and you could never be as interesting as this gif.'

This feels particularly prominent in big cities where everyone seems to have that air of busyness and importance around them, which is palpably dismantled in areas where the pace of life is slower and arguably more comfortable, and everyone's keen for a chat – like more regional suburbs, or the entirety of Wales.

Of course, if you have depression, you feel completely worthless anyway, so it's even more excruciatingly difficult to have the confidence to make a friend or try to open yourself up to anyone at all, because you're utterly convinced that you're not enough and have nothing to offer. If you're anything like me you've probably found yourself wondering why anyone would want to spend time with you, when you might cancel plans, cry at any moment, be totally silent and not have anything to say, or just brush people off all the time in favour of being alone.

Why would anyone want to be friends with you in the first place?

When your brain has been wired to tell you that you're worthless and that everything you do or think is wrong, it's gonna be hard to speak to new people – hell, it's hard to speak to your mum – and you've heard how horrible you are when you speak to yourself.

As someone trying to talk themselves out of self-loathing on the daily, I'm not quite yet at the place where I can tell you how to overcome this worthlessness because I definitely haven't got there myself. BUT, luckily I've been 'on the emails' with Kate

Mason from Roots Psychology Group, who has actual qualified opinions and speaks a lot of sense. She has the answers that I don't have (and, if I may say, quite the breathtakingly beautiful and powerful first name):

> *Depression is like having a bully sitting on your shoulder every day, telling you that you are worthless and no good. If this was a real-life person we may choose to distance ourselves from that person (or maybe tell them what we think!) but we can't escape this 'depression bully'.*

> *If someone tells you over and over every day that you are worthless, then eventually you start to believe it. The good news is that with some self-discipline we can adopt a few strategies to begin to help ourselves emerge from the fog.*

I think it's important here to highlight something that I'm still struggling to come to terms with, but that is (allegedly) essential for me and any other depressed person to acknowledge:

You are not worthless. The depression demons are in your brain and are tricking you into feeling this way. You are not an unlovable, pointless collection of cells and don't let the damn demons make you think that you are.

It's hard to get your head around that bit, though, isn't it? Somebody once kept telling me, 'You would be fine if you just stopped hating yourself so much.' Yeah, no shit. I'd LOVE to not hate myself. I want the confidence of Beyoncé on stage at Coachella, or of a mediocre straight white man in a meeting. I want to love myself as much as I love others. It's not that easy, though, is it?

Kate Mason has some more qualified, professional advice,

which I'm all ready to try to follow because I still think of myself as a human turd.

Join me, fellow turd-feeler:

Quieten your inner critic. When your inner critic tells you over and over that you are not good enough, you start to believe it. When this happens, try to slow yourself down and ask yourself, 'What are the facts here and what is just my inner critic throwing inaccurate ideas into the mix?'

Work on reducing negative self-talk. Identifying your strengths can help dampen that self-hatred. If you find it difficult to come up with some on your own, consider asking others for help. It is almost always easier to recognize some else's strengths rather than our own.

Develop self-compassion. People who struggle with self-hatred often have little or no compassion towards themselves. A great way to think of self-compassion is to think about how you would treat a friend or loved one, and treat yourself the same. No one has ever said we have to be perfect – learn to give yourself a break, ask yourself, 'What would I say to my ten-year-old self?' Would you tell them off for not being perfect?

Learn to accept compliments. If you view yourself in a hateful way, it's hard to take a compliment. It may feel awkward and uncomfortable so we tend to dismiss it or minimize it to avoid feeling vulnerable. It takes practice but give it a go – the next time someone compliments you, try saying 'thank you' – and stop there. Resist the urge to follow it up with a self-critical or dismissive response.

'Self-hatred is often focused on the past – a painful moment or emotion like shame or guilt, anger or embarrassment, or a sense of powerlessness,' Kate told me. 'Try and focus on the present and remind yourself how far you've come since then. It may well feel strange at first, but over time it will help you gain that self-compassion.

'Stopping self-hatred takes time, but as you allow yourself to let go of the negative critic, you make room for more joy, peace, and connection in your life.'

Anyway, we were travelling down this murky road of self-hatred because the existence of such loathing puts up something of a barrier when we think about trying to get strangers to like us.

Look at all the lonely people (and run away)

If the whole concept of making new real-life friends seems as likely as Leonardo DiCaprio dating someone his own age, you of course shouldn't feel obliged to be signing up to clubs, thinking of fake hobbies you could just about tolerate and joining a local riot group to start making protest signs on the back of your old cereal boxes.

Depression mixes itself up into a different, delightful recipe of fuckery for everyone, and in my case it came with a healthy dollop of social anxiety, too. This was a fun game! I could fake it at work in front of a conference room full of suits, but couldn't face seeing people that I knew really, really well in a pub down the road. Absolute bants! You can decide to quit your job and navigate Central America on your own, but you can't be alone in your lovely flat because you'll hyperventilate and then get sick! Ah, the thrills of a contradictory mental illness.

I think this kind of depression facade is the same kind of fight or flight reaction that's triggered in us when we're carrying a really hot drink to a table; we know it's burning our hand, but we also know if we drop it then it'll be a faff to clean up and there'll be china and scorching tea all over the floor and we'll probably ruin our jeans. So, we keep holding the mug and keep slowly burning our hand because in the long run that's just better than cleaning up the mess.

Depression is the burning inside of us that we grit our teeth and smile through, because admitting that it burns would cause such a hot mess that it wouldn't be worth trying to clean up afterwards, and we'd wish we'd just carried on pretending everything was fine. Right?

I knew it was probably time to seek out some help when the process of getting ready to attend someone's birthday curry sent me into a fit of hyperventilation and sweating, followed by a small vomit. A curry somewhere reasonably cheap and comfy in Camden with people that I see regularly made me crawl into bed and hide under the duvet like a child, waiting for the coast to be clear and the monster to go away. But the monster doesn't go away when it's in your head, does it?

This is a whole new side order of crap to accompany the well of darkness. We know how important friendship and company (even silent company – actually, sometimes *especially* silent company) are. Actual science has proved that expressions of friendship can help change our brain chemistry and HEY, isn't that what we're all looking for through our bleak landscapes of serotonin deprivation?[25]

Having a long hug (twenty seconds or longer – yeah, it might seem a bit weird and get awkward around the eight-second mark, but listen to the science) releases oxytocin, and honestly, I'm willing to do anything that can shoot a little goodness into my brain.

In a non-scientific but potentially still notable observation, I find the 'cuddle hormone' to also be particularly strong when people take MDMA, but you're not best advised to shuck a few bombs before your team-building afternoon of trust-falls.

Robot friends

We're the generation that grew up with AIM and MSN Messenger, where conversations seemed achingly intimate on the privacy of a computer screen and after curfew. We shared little pieces of our feelings via overly dramatic screen names, and expressed our totally edgy identities by using song lyrics or jokes as our statuses, and picking a font and text colour that perfectly summed us up. I legitimately remember telling someone after they changed their font on MSN Messenger that 'this feels weird, it doesn't feel like I'm talking to you anymore'. The absolute cringe of it all.

But this penchant for messaging has made us allergic to phone calls. We'll book restaurants through apps to avoid speaking to someone, make a haircut appointment online to swerve any voice action and book bikini waxes on an app to avoid speaking on the phone to someone to whom we will willingly display our hairy labia. Once we get into our taxi that we voicelessly ordered through our phones, we can even choose 'quiet preferred' mode to stop any possible interactions with the human Uber driver.

We are sending voice notes, but not making phone calls. We

are talking to our freaky AI house-robots and asking them to play some music or to find a fact online, but we're not making phone calls. We'll have a group chat about going for Sunday lunch that is forty-seven messages long, but we won't make a phone call.

Harvard Business Review (yeah, I read that stuff) published a study that showed a face-to-face interaction is thirty-four times more impactful than a text interaction when it comes to asking for donations or attendance or something like that,[26] but don't you think it's a similar impact when you're just saying hi, checking in, asking about lunch or a coffee, or wishing someone a happy birthday?

All of this was completely out of reach when I was sinking, though. There's no way I'd actually *call* someone to say I wasn't coming out, I'd always cop out with a text message and an appropriate, carefully selected emoji – then nobody has to hear the cracks in my voice or notice that I'm crying. If someone called me I would always, *always* screen, and voicemails would pile up unlistened to because I couldn't stand the guilt of having ignored them in the first place. Social anxiety will kick you in the back of the knees when you least expect it and pull you out of situations that used to be so mundane and normal, turning them into unimaginable horrors.

As a person who once hyperventilated on the number 73 bus when some 'impromptu plans' were announced by my ex-boyfriend (said plans: going to meet three friends in a pub nearby), I'm in no position to offer counsel or advice, really. Luckily, Kate Mason has come through once again with all her helpful qualifications and opinions and wisdom.

I asked her for her thoughts about social anxiety, and why

we get so fearful of people even when we know, love and trust them. She assured me that social anxiety, like most things in this book, is NOT YOUR FAULT so stop blaming yourself for being a pansy when the thought of a group dinner is making you want to dig a burrow and hide in it forever. 'There's actually something going on in your brain when this happens,' Kate told me. 'If you are socially anxious, you see people and social encounters as a threat, therefore your brain goes into fight or flight mode and you become focused on keeping yourself safe and alive.

'As a result, the part of our brain that's responsible for actually being sociable (the executive functioning that takes place around the judging panel) essentially shuts down – so skills like reasoning, negotiation, forward thinking, recognizing social etiquette and impulse control – i.e. all the clever skills that enable us to hold a conversation – shut off, as your brain is telling you "hang on, love, you need to get the hell outta there"'.

So, see, it's really not you, it's your brain plagued with social anxiety demons and the other fun spoils of depression. Hmm, not sure if that's actually good news or not.

Depression gets in the way of plans that you might even be looking forward to, and doesn't give a hoot about how long you haven't seen someone for if it's trying to convince you to stay in and hide. The most useful advice I've had around this is to really look at your phone calendar (or paper diary if you like to keep things romantic) and block out time for when you know you'll probably be feeling drained. For example, if I have dinner with friends one night, the next day I'm likely to feel exhausted from the performative conversation and want to do nothing but retreat. So I'll block this day out, and won't make any social plans that may end up being cancelled at the last minute.

Panic! at the disco. Freak out! in the pub

While this is a genuinely useful strategy, there are also the events planned so far in advance that they become overly hyped and then ripe for being a total let-down. This of course applies to non-depressed people too (apparently they exist?) and New Year's Eve is undoubtedly the worst of the lot.

So what do we do when we've promised attendance to something important (if not to us, then to others) and then, when the time comes around, the thought of trying to prise yourself out of your misery is too exhausting and disintegrating to bear? I haven't the foggiest, but award-winning psychologist Natasha Tiwari (founder of The Veda Group, a global wellness advisery company), does:

> *You need to remind yourself that you wouldn't punish your-*
> *self for feeling the need to cancel if you were physically weak*
> *or in poor physical health, and that if the shoe was on the*
> *other foot, you wouldn't hesitate to show your friend the*
> *same compassion that you deserve in this moment. Allow*
> *yourself that compassion.*

> *Know that you're not doing anything wrong, and trust that*
> *your friend cares enough about you that they won't take*
> *your need for rest as an insult. Tell your friend honestly the*
> *truth of your mood and how it's affecting you, how you so*

appreciate their patience and still being invited despite not being 'on form'.

You may find yourself surprised at how your friendship deepens as a result of your sharing so honestly.

Making more succinct plans with a select group of people – or often only individuals – was a slow step back in for me. Lunches or quick coffees worked well as you could feign other following commitments that you had to run off to. For a while I thought the cinema would be good as we wouldn't actually have to talk, but it seems that the moment you're submerged in darkness and your brain thinks nobody can see you, it's impossible to stop the tears from falling. Quite awkward at the 2 p.m. Sunday screening of *Finding Dory*.

Let's take a moment here, because all this advice and #relatable-content is great (right? RIGHT?) but what about when you're so heavily into the mind-tar that leaving the house is barely tolerable at best, and you've isolated yourself to the extent that you're a bit of a Billy-no-mates these days. How in Peggy Mitchell's name do you actually make friends when you're above the age of eleven? Forging new relationships is *hard*; most people are either coupled off, already have their own friendship groups and don't need new friends or think you're a twat.

The whole 'Just join a club! You'll make friends instantly!' trope is tired, but true. Clichés tend to be clichés because they work, not because they're a bag of lies set up to trick you. Time DOES help heal. The grass IS always greener on the other side. Too many cooks DO spoil the broth and joining a club CAN actually help you make friends, dammit.

Some psychologists have said that to form friendships you must have repeated interactions (duh) and share a common interest. As a person with a job and a brain that's on fire, it's hard to keep appointments with friends – but if those friends will be somewhere you're gonna go anyway every Wednesday evening, it's much easier to stick to the plans.

Also, most other people who joined this club or group are there for exactly the same reason as you are. They feel a bit low on the friends supply and they're looking for something fun to do where they can meet people who hopefully won't murder them in their sleep.

In the spirit of trying to be helpful, behold some actual ways in which actual people have made new friends when they were out in the wild. No freshers' weeks, speed dating or 'I sat next to her at work!' allowed.

- 'I decided to become vegan, and started posting about it on Instagram to keep me motivated. I soon found a vegan community and connected with other Instagrammers from my area. Now we meet up to try new vegan places or menu options. I realize this sounds totally naff, but I didn't intend to make friends like this. It just happened.'
- 'I found my main circle of friends by becoming mates with my boyfriend's sister. We got on so well and she started to invite me out with her friends. Now, even though my boyfriend and I split up five years ago, we're still a really tight group of girls.'
- 'I became a volunteer at Girl Guiding, and have made three really good new friends in the past year because of it. We all went to Sweden this summer with twenty-five Girl Guides

– it was great.' (This sounds like my personal version of hell, but if you have a warmer soul than me I guess it would be a good shout.)

- 'I went along to a local protest about puppies being sold at a local pet shop. It was attended by a completely different set of people than I'd normally hang out with, and we became friends through regular protests and meetings to stop third-party puppy sales. We even got Michael Gove to introduce #LucysLaw because of it.'

- (Forgive this next contributor for she is American…) 'I made friends at an Aaron Carter concert when I saw people holding a sign that said *"Aaron we saw you in 2002 and you wore shiny silver pants"* with a drawing of the pants. We talked and laughed about the sign and ended up watching the concert together and exchanging Facebook details before we left. This led to chatting and exchanging phone numbers, and now we truly are close friends.'

- 'I felt lonely AF when I moved to London, so looked for a mixed-gender sport I could sign up to on my own so I could make friends. I found tag rugby, and now those people are my main social group. We have pub visits every week and lots of dinners.'

- 'I joined some classes at my local gym, and after a few weeks of seeing the same people every week we started to have some chats. Conversation would be about how hungover we were or how hard we found the class, etc., and we ended up swapping social media details. Now we hang out all the time.'

- 'I found a local university that was running "taster sessions" of evening classes, so I went along to a creative writing session. I was nervous asking if anyone wanted to go for a glass of wine afterwards and talk about their ideas, but it seemed like everyone was there both to write *and* make friends, so there were takers straight away.'

- 'I joined a rugby club that was set up for people who had never played before, so everyone there was in the same boat. We trained for six weeks and then played our first match together, and it was a real bonding experience.'

Ugh, tired ol' clichés amiright? But the beauty of this bastard internet that we all live our lives on is that we can search for local clubs and events that are designed for clueless beginners, so there's no chance of accidentally signing up to an expert fencing club and having to leave after ten minutes because everyone's a bit too advanced with their swordsmanship.

Also, I like what the creative writing person said about being nervous to ask people for a drink before remembering that everyone there probably quite wanted to be asked for a drink, really. It's intimidating asking strangers if they want to go and socialize with you, but the likely outcome is that most other people in the class have joined said class as a way of meeting people, because otherwise they'd just stay home and take a class on the goddam internet —YouTube tutorials are free and don't involve speaking to anyone (but weirdly all seem to involve the narrator person doing a lot of heavy breathing. Why?), so anyone who's chosen to actually leave the house and attend a class is probably up for a bit of IRL interaction. Plus, if they say no you're still the same friendless loner you were before, so you've got nothing to lose.

A friend in need is a friend indeed – or are they just super annoying?

So, OK, you put this book down and spent a month joining classes and you've made some weird pottery things and are learning to play the ukulele, and now you and your new friend Alex have seen each other most weekends and you're WhatsApping more and more and sharing 'So us!' posts on Instagram. Yahoo for you. But what happens now, when… oh God, what happens if Alex finds out that you're secretly a fucking miserable depressed demon?

Introducing someone to your depression is like revealing you have a gangrenous third leg: it's always been there, but you're not exactly gonna lead with it on a first meeting. You can cover up your messed-up third leg with clever clothing, by only meeting on the 'good leg days' or by choosing activities that mean it won't fly out of your gusset. You can hide it for a fair whack of time but at some point you're gonna have to say, 'Listen, mate, I can't come out tonight because I need to tend to my third leg' – or trip over it in public, more likely.

Then comes the part when your manky leg's out, you're both looking at it, and you most likely try to laugh it off as something that never usually happens – but it does. Your wasting, souring third leg isn't going anywhere and the time to address it is now. What happens next is a little muddier (as if this third-leg analogy wasn't razor sharp already…).

Illness isn't classist, racist or homophobic. Hopefully your new pal (or, even trickier, date… gulp) is aware of this and understanding of the fact that you've slapped a bandage on it for the few times you've hung out before. But if things are moving to a more frequent schedule – even if it's just more messages or meme-sharing – then sometimes you might not be fully functional because your goddam leg is giving you jip.

'Let's go back to how it was before' is one of the most cutting responses I've had to this, a few months into a new friendship with someone and after I'd opened up about my mental fuckery. I was having a particularly bad week with it, and being fairly mute. 'We don't talk like we used to' and 'I feel like you're avoiding me' are both acceptable viewpoints or responses, but they're indicative that this person absolutely does not understand what you're going through and either needs to be more informed, if you both want this relationship to be something that works, or needs to be phased out if you can't be bothered with more comments that make you feel guilty for not being a constant hoot.

They were phased out.

One of the absolute worst things this friend used to say to me (until I told him to please, please stop) was 'I just want to see you smile'. Sure, it sounds innocent and of course I love it when the people I love are happy – who doesn't love to see a friend smiling? – but whenever he said it to me it felt like a tsunami of pressure to 'just be happy', or at least just to fake it, for him. I too would like to see myself (genuinely) smile more often; I don't revel in my misery and wake up every morning doing a little fist pump that nothing has changed and I still feel dark. I want to be one of those people with unmarked brains who can smile all the time too. Believe me.

Depression is more than a mental illness, though, and can manifest in truly horrible physical symptoms and urges. One of the most common is an urge to self-harm, which, if you go ahead with it, of course leaves physical scarring alongside the mental. These marks are the 'manky leg' analogy brought to life, as there'll usually come a point when it's too hot to wear long sleeves or trousers, and then what do you do when your scars are revealed in all their shiny, warped-tissue glory, when everyone's just trying to have a few cans in the park on a hot day?

Thinking of telling anyone about your mental health can be intimidating. Even in this modern age of streaming and Deliveroo (what a time to be alive and want to die) when we're all encouraging each other to 'speak up and reach out' (gag), it remains a sensitive subject. My tale of casually mentioning it to Dré in bed is just one flakey story. Here are some others:

- 'The first person I spoke to was my best friend. She knew for a long time something was up but I would bat away any speculation, meaning she felt that she couldn't get through. Once I explained everything to her, I felt both extremely lost, like there was no escape, yet calm, like there was nothing left in me. Now that I've worked hard on my mental health, I'm in a place where I can stay on top of things and recognize the signs before it gets to the point of no return.'

- 'I told my boyfriend. I felt anxious about telling him because I didn't want him to see me differently. Since I've been taking the medication and have told him, our communication is much more open and it feels so good to be honest with him.'

- 'I was obviously nervous before I told anyone, but by being honest with my nearest and dearest, it felt like a big relief and weight off my shoulders. There was a period of feeling anxious about how they would take it and that they would think I was crazy, but I believe that is the depression talking rather than what they actually think about me.'

- 'It's a part of my therapy to be very open about it because otherwise I feel like I'm keeping a deep dark secret that eats at me. I don't feel anything in particular prior to telling people, but I always feel relieved when I do.'

- 'Recently I had to inform my workplace, specifically my managers, about my depression and how it can impact me. All in all, telling them felt just like the sensation of chewing cotton wool. Nothing I said felt right, despite having looked up every shred of information over the years on how to inform people, as well as having a strong history of being open with friends about mental health. I felt as though I was constantly trying to balance between being completely honest about the intensity of my depression, and trying not to say anything of the sort for fear if I did, I'd lose my job or be seen as incapable. Although they were understanding, I felt as though telling them placed a large space between us; as though I'd alienated myself. Afterwards, I felt pressure to act "normal", to prove that I could work well.'

- 'I told my work recently after having to take several weeks off. I feel like it has given me some confidence back, and that I'm no longer living under a shadow.'

- 'I've suffered with depression my whole life. The first time I told my mum I broke down in my car. I didn't really have a choice about telling her, it all just came out. It's always been a bit of a sign of weakness for me, so normally I just go on until I burst into tears. So much drama.'

- 'A few times I've mentioned it to friends – there had been alcoholic beverages involved. These times were easy – afterwards (the next day) I felt indifferent about it. When I told someone sober, beforehand I felt ashamed, awkward and stupid… like, there were no major problems in my life, I have no reason to feel the way I do. Afterwards, I felt like I could breathe.'

- 'The first person I told was my boyfriend. Before doing so, I felt a great sense of shame, like I had "failed" in some way or was broken. His response was overwhelmingly supportive and positive and the guilt of my sadness didn't feel as heavy anymore. I have gone on to tell lots and lots of people now – I hope that it might help someone else who is in a dark place to speak up.'

When I was asking people to tell me how they've spoken to others about their mental health, there were only a handful of people who actually had. A lot of people I spoke to said they were too apprehensive to talk about it as they worried their friends and family would 'just think they were attention seeking', which is an awful thing to worry about, and I like to think that no family would react in that way… but you never know.

If you don't want to just call your pal an attention-seeking drama queen and actually do want to help them or support them as they're going through depression, here are some things you might wanna try:

- Keep inviting them to things. Even if they always say no or cancel at the last minute, keep them included.
- Spend time 'together' online. My glorious sister and I often watch a Netflix show together from our own separate sofas and houses (there are apps that make this easier, or you can

just text each other 'three, two, one, go'). It's a lovely way of feeling like you have company and support and equally being a blubbering mess on your own. Thanks, sister.

- Try to spend one-on-one time with them. A great way to do this is to invite them to join something you'd already be doing anyway, like going to a café or opening the biscuits you bought when you were hungry in aisle five, or going for a walk. My best friend Tom has previously invited me to his place to watch a film and not talk to each other, so we could be alone together. It was and always is perfect. Thanks, Tom.

- Know that you cannot fix them. Don't tell them about things you read online or suggest things that might make them feel better. Just be there for them.

- Understand that 'being there' for them doesn't mean waiting for them to get in touch. Check in – but in a casual way, not in a 'Sooo… offed yourself yet?' way. Actually, that might get a chuckle.

- Tag them in memes. Honestly, in this modern world there is no better compliment than someone thinking of you when they see something they liked.

- Understand that they have no control over it. Depression fog is like real fog; sometimes there's none at all, sometimes you can't see.

- Remember that they're probably doing all they can to push through it. Just because they're dressed and out with you doesn't mean they're not depressed that particular day, it means they're trying to swim up for air.

- Know that there's probably nothing you can say that will help. At all. But continuing to hang around will be immense, even when they're a miserable twat.

I asked some people what it feels like to be on the other side, to be told that someone you care about is depressed. Spoiler alert, nobody said, 'Ugh, it made me want them out of my life IMMEDIATELY, WHAT A FREAK,' and everyone was understanding. The general gist is, much like Dré said, that it made the person on the receiving end more understanding of the depressed person's behaviours, and actually much less likely to think that they're a twat.

- 'I was glad they told me. I looked at their behaviour and realized that some of the things I may have judged them for were symptoms of their illness. It has meant we have a more open and honest relationship.'
- 'I really appreciated being told. I have a friend who doesn't talk a lot about her personal life and for her to finally open up to me was a big deal. It gave us more space to talk about feelings now that I know she's not OK sometimes.'
- 'I feel grateful for my friend to have opened up about his depression. Our relationship feels closer.'
- 'I feel touched that they trust me enough to open up with me, but it doesn't change our relationship any more than the person wants it to change our relationship – some friends don't want to bring it up often and others appreciate regular check-ins.'

See?

If you're on the receiving end and someone you care about has just told you that they're depressed, my advice is to listen. 'I had no idea you were struggling, how are you feeling/tell me what it's like for you?' is a great start. Asking what you can do to help seems kind but realistically you won't get an answer, as it's likely that your friend either doesn't know what they need, or doesn't want to be a burden – or both. Listening to them tell you about how they feel and if they are making any plans to try to manage the illness is kind and supportive. You can always ask if they notice anything in particular that makes them feel better or worse, but your main job here is to listen, hug and let them know that you're around for them. Keep inviting them. Keep checking in. Keep listening.

The clapbacks

If someone is suggesting that you make new friends, it probably comes from a place of kindness (unless they're suggesting it so you end up hanging out with them less...) and maybe they just need to understand how you feel.

> 'I'm not lonely, I spend a lot of time alone because I need the people who *are* in my life to be more understanding of what's going on in my head. Here, why don't you read this great book...'

> 'I'm finding it hard to be my own friend right now, so I'm hardly ready to bring this onto new people.'

> 'I want to. Show me how. Come with me. Be my friend.'

CHAPTER 8

You should look after yourself more, honey

We've reached a point now where the definitions are very blurry around what constitutes 'self-care' and what is actually just doing a face mask and bunking off work. Self-care is essentially defined as looking after your daily functional needs: eating, sleeping and hygiene, but has now become so bastardized by the internet that people will chalk absolutely anything up to 'self-care', from a £400 spa day to a pint of Baileys in the bath (would absolutely recommend the latter, for what it's worth).

There's a difference between genuinely cancelling plans because you feel like you want to kill yourself and would rather be at home drinking red wine straight from the bottle, and cancelling plans because you can't be arsed to go out. Technology (ooh, is this *Black Mirror*?) has now made us all little flakes who cancel on friends forty-five minutes before we're due to hang out, and it's largely put down to the fact that we need some time for self-care.

Actual, basic self-care can seem wildly out of reach when you're living with depression (as we remember from my boybander experience near the croissants). Looking after yourself isn't high on your priorities list, because what's the point? Things can't get any worse, surely, so you might as well let yourself go. Why book a haircut when you know full well you're not going to be able to get out of bed for a week? Why go grocery shopping when your appetite is so weird, and why take a shower when you're not going to see anyone else anyway? I think 'non-depressed people' experienced this during the coronavirus lockdown, which has actually served as a useful way to reference this effect of your depression. 'It's like being on lockdown but all the time' is now bitterly relatable.

There is, of course, a scientific reason for this, and it's all to do with the frontal lobe in your brain.

Research shows that when you're depressed the frontal lobe begins to dysfunction, so your judgement and decision making goes absolutely out the window, and looking after yourself has been long forgotten. You have no attention span or willpower, and it's a struggle to remember what you were doing a few hours ago. No wonder you look like crap.

The frontal lobe (the left and right frontal cortexes, if we're going to get specific) are also crucial for empathy, so it makes sense that when you're depressed you largely feel a numbness and are lacking in reactions to just about anything.

But it's fine! Just do a face mask!

Face masks don't work when you're crying.

Alas, the current facemask market doesn't offer a bee-pollen-and-local-seaweed treatment that magically gets rid of intrusive thoughts, but there is definitely some value in taking a moment to look after yourself – no matter how worthless you feel.

Millennials have been heralded (yup, a good thing) as being obsessed with self-care,[27] which actually ties in with us also being spoken of as the generation with the most emotional intelligence, because we know that self-care is hugely important when we're alive in a world that's metaphorically and physically on fire. Well done, us.

Our generation is frantic; there's a lot going on in our minds. We're swallowing enormous student debts and looking at a job market more competitive than Texan children's beauty pageants. We're busting our asses in jobs when we do eventually land them, and we likely don't have a pension or any savings – but hey, the world will soon be on fire anyway, so what are we even saving for?

We've reached a level of burnout that is staggering and isn't the result of us being feeble little snowflakes. Yes, there was a hefty chunk of people that didn't exactly help the cause by complaining viciously about the struggle of 'adulting' (performing everyday basic tasks that we need to do in order to live a modern life, i.e. go to work, pay bills and taxes, clean things and do paperwork). The vernacular doesn't do a lot to legitimize the concerns here but getting to a point where your brain is so fried and your body is so wired that you can't perform even simple tasks is very real.

But to realize that you might need to start taking *more* care of yourself implies that you're someone who takes even a tiny bit of care of yourself in the first place. When every time you wake up in the morning you feel a gut-punch at the thought of trying to get through the day ahead, it's hard to think about the long term.

It's impossible to plan a 'career trajectory' when the thought of still being here and feeling like this long enough to see it play out is the worst-case scenario. It's ridiculous looking for a decent rental flat contract when you want to double over at the thought of *still being here and feeling like this* when it starts.

To be able to give yourself care, you need to have self-awareness, which doesn't come easily when you're depressed. Being cognizant of your specific needs and weaknesses is quite a feat when you generally have one large need to lie in the darkness and cry until you fall into the sweet, unconscious world of sleep. You cannot think of doing something that will make yourself feel better in the immediate or near future, because all you can think about is the giant rope around your waist pulling you further and further down, right now. All you can feel is a gloomy fog billowing around your empty insides, and it's got no chance of lifting anytime soon.

Depression sucks our energy away, and if you're running on fumes then you're going to focus on only getting the essentials done to make it through another painful day. Self-care doesn't usually make it to those priorities.

We know by now that depression has a huge effect on the brain's hippocampus, and that that part of the brain is responsible for most of our 'executive decisions', and is essentially host to the judging panel of our life. When that plays host to the depression demons, though, it's harder for the judging panel to think about the future *at all*, from the 'what do you want to be when you grow up?' to the 'how are you going to get home tonight?' options. It's so shrouded in life-suckers that our ability to imagine the future impact of anything is pretty much totally mangled. So yeah, don't blame yourself if brushing your hair or having a bath is overdue, blame the depression demons.

Depression kicks the desks over in the parts of your brain responsible for decision making and forward planning,[28] and depression ruins your ability to think sharply, to make decisions comfortably and to remember things clearly.[29] Lo and behold, you can't really imagine future things clearly, either. Fun!

Think about the Depression Bully sitting on your shoulder that Kate Mason described (fuck that bully): 'We need to work out a way to separate us from the bully and that involves becoming self-aware. Depression feels like a blanket smothering us to the point we don't know what's real anymore, so our senses can be numbed.'

Why would you want to care for something – or someone – you hate? When your opinion of yourself is as low as it gets (thinking you should be dead really is the lowest opinion of yourself you can have, guys, you can't get worse than that, well done, everyone – see, we *are* achievers) then you're hardly going to want to give yourself water and sunshine so your leaves grow. Self-care is about looking after the self you already are, right? When your current self is the Mayor of Doomsville, cultivating that self doesn't seem like such a great idea.

When we feel overwhelmed (or like death), seemingly self-indulgent activities (that are really just basic needs and functions) will be the first things to go. How many times have you missed a meal because you were too busy? Or waited to finish a bit of work before you 'rewarded' yourself by going to the bathroom? Or – be honest here – taken clothes out of the dirty laundry basket to re-wear them because you don't have time to put a wash on?

Self-care has to be given to you *by you*, and if you're not feeling up to even facing the day let alone providing yourself with an at-home-spa treatment, you're really not alone.

Kate Mason reminded me that self-care doesn't have to involve pricey spas or weekends away in the countryside:

We need to be able to take care of ourselves in the moment: at home, at work, in the car, in the supermarket, or out with family and friends. This is about not looking out into the environment for something to make us feel better, it's about having what we call an 'internal locus of control', i.e. working on your own ability to manage your mood and increase self-awareness.

Recognizing when we're feeling particularly doomful, and perhaps trying to work out if there's something specific that's enhancing the doom, can start with noticing how you feel, both physically and emotionally, by paying closer attention to what is happening in your body so that you can gather an idea of what's going on in your mind. Noticing symptoms early means you can do something about it before it turns into a full-blown episode.

For me, there are a few things that I know will make me feel more exhausted and low, and when I feel myself starting to descend it's usually because of one of the following:

- I'm about a week away from getting my period and the hormone cocktail has made my depression more severe.
- I haven't been getting enough sleep.
- I've had a few social occasions in a row and not much alone time.
- Conversely, I've been alone too long and haven't had any meaningful affection.
- I've been drinking too much.

The warning signs usually start in my chest, which feels like it's being crushed by a medieval jouster. I'll notice that I'm crankier than usual and getting annoyed by everything, and that my eyes are always teared up. If I take a few minutes to think about what I've been doing lately, it's usually an indicator that I've not been too kind to myself and that I'm about to host the depression demons for a while. Kate says:

> Ask yourself, 'What am I feeling here and where do I feel it?' Take some deep breaths and breathe into the areas of your body where you can feel it. Deep breathing increases circulation, releases endorphins and relaxes muscles.

Really, if you're at the point where 'self-care' is just surviving, don't feel pressured to do a ten-step exfoliation routine before a hammam spa and hot mud wrap. 'To keep breathing' is enough to aim for. Plus, caring for yourself can be as much about *not* doing something as it can be about purposefully taking action to do something.

A huge study involving 10,000 patients was published in 2018, and confirmed that the brains of people with depression are set up to think they're pieces of crap.[30] 'In the brains of those living with depressive problems, they discovered a strong connection between the dorsolateral prefrontal cortex (associated with short-term memory), the precuneus (associated with the self) and the lateral orbitofrontal cortex (associated with negative emotion).' So basically, your brain's connections have fixed themselves into a structure that tells you that you are worth nothing, and that's all you can remember in the short term. LOLs!

I'm not quite at the stage where I think I'm worth much just yet, so for me a lot of the 'taking care of yourself' stuff comes down to me knowing my limits and knowing when to say no. It's about knowing that I need a lot of time on my own, and that spending too much time with other people will exhaust me and make me feel angry and irritable. It's also about knowing that sometimes when I've had too much time alone I can be energized by the company of, and conversation with, a close friend, even if it's just over the phone. This self-awareness stuff has a lot going for it, really. So does putting everything into your phone's calendar app so you can keep track.

My version of self-care is to try to stop blaming myself for being depressed, and stop apologizing for it. Yes, depression played a huge part in the end of my relationship and I'm truly sorry that Dré had to live with someone who was trying to cover up how miserable they were and that the magnitude of the depression was too encompassing and staggering to be able to avoid, in the end. But I'm not sorry I'm depressed. Yes, I hate it, but I didn't *choose* it. Saying sorry for having depression is like saying sorry for having an enormous chest; you might hate it and try to cover it and distract attention far, far away from it, but you didn't go to a shop and choose it and say, 'Ooh yes, that fits nicely, I'll take it!' – it's out of your control.

But, acknowledging that you have it and that you need to consciously work with it and around it is really most of what we can do. By reading this very book you've already done that, so HURRAH, well done you. Like someone accepting their enormous breasts and finally caving in and buying an ugly but oh-so-supportive bra to help with their back pain, realizing that you need to manage your depression can also have an instantaneous effect (and, isn't it nice to compare depression to some big, jiggling breasts?).

Some things I do that feel nice when I feel horrible that I suggest you try yourself within the next twenty minutes:

- Exfoliate your face because, oh man, it feels amazing. Then moisturize it.
- Get one of those head massagers that looks like a metal spider. So good.
- Watch *Die Hard*.
- Remember an album that you used to love, turn off your phone and listen to the entire thing from start to finish while doing nothing else.
- Nap.
- Get a tennis ball or a hard apple and roll your foot around on top of it for a strange body massage that zings up your leg (try it, I promise).
- Eat ice cream.
- Treat yourself like you would a dog: call it cute, give it treats, make sure it gets plenty of naps and opportunities for lovely walks.

Welcome to the stage: Mariah self-Carey

So how can you be self-caring without being self-sabotaging? And what constitutes self-care and what's just you being lazy and rude?

Look at it as self-preservation, rather than self-indulgence, and remember the power of saying a hard nope. I've tried to start by not blaming myself for how my depression impacts me and everyone else. Yeah, it sucks, but it's not my fault I'm depressed.

According to Instagram's more than 30 million #selfcare posts, self-care is all about drinking mugs of herbal tea on bougie table settings, and getting a new head of highlights at the salon. According to me, self-care is about taking off the pressure and allowing yourself to just be. Just BE. Pay attention to how you're feeling and what you're thinking and let the thoughts and feelings flood into you and don't blame yourself for their existence.

The whole concept of self-care is now a commercialized hell-fest, with 'self-care kits' being sold due to the cutesy slogans on their sleeping masks and positive affirmations on the miniature calendars. Social media's self-care is about thick whipped cream on a velvety hot chocolate, or a floating dinner tray holding your glistening cheesy pizza while you're in the bath. To me, the real concept of self-care is looking after your brain hygiene just as you would your dental hygiene, but that's not quite as clickable or sellable, is it?

Kate Mason has some non-ridiculous advice for the self-loathing who are trying to move into self-awareness, and thus, self-care. She is 100% That Bitch.[31] She told me:

> *Try to notice what you're telling yourself. We say negative things to ourselves all the time, like a record on repeat telling you you're not good enough, that you're unlovable, stupid, and should have done that better. Our feelings of*

guilt, shame and negative thoughts all influence how we speak to ourselves. You could be loved by everyone and be as successful as Bill Gates, but the strength of self-talk will always be more powerful.

A thing to try to see if you can be nice to yourself

Kate Mason suggests, 'As an exercise, try writing down some of the horrible things you tell yourself.

'Now look at the list, call your best mate and tell them that THEY are all those things.

'OK, please don't. Would you really say any of those things to your friend? My guess is no, so why say it to yourself? **Your mind only hears what you tell it** so try to notice when you're being hard on yourself and practise some compassion.

'Notice how often you put yourself down or scrutinize your behaviour, then challenge these statements. Depression tells you that you are rubbish in every aspect of your life – in relationships, in your abilities, at work , everywhere – so try to write down something you DO like about yourself, even if you don't fully believe it. Repeat it like a mantra to yourself; if this feels weird adopt the "fake it til you feel it" idea until you begin to change your mindset.'

We know that depression has messed up our frontal lobe, and the demons looming around our judging panel are sucking away their ability to judge anything at all, to make future plans or to pay much attention to what's happening right now. Start small. Reading a magnificent book such as this is a great step, as it shows you have the self-awareness to realize that, yup, you are depressed and, yup, it's horrible and, yup, you want to be able to do something about it. But what?

During the times I'm so dark I stay in bed the whole time, a huge achievement can be just sitting up in bed. Even bigger can be turning the lamp on, and even more insurmountable still might be to put on some mindless television, music, radio or noise that you don't have to think about and that can be controlled from your bedside table. Thank you, technology.

Action is hard when your brain is on fire, but the thing about the brain is that it's malleable. It's changeable, and we can coax it into other presentations where it isn't aflame and our judging panel aren't on their last legs – we just have to exercise it into that state, and trying to turn its focus onto one pleasant thing can help. Maybe it's getting into a bed with freshly washed sheets, and as you sink under the covers you can concentrate on deeply inhaling the smell. Maybe it's opening the curtain just a crack, so you can look at the slice of light and perhaps even feel a line of warmth on your body where the sun lands.

Look, I'm not a self-help guru, and my experiences won't be the same as your experiences, so here are a bunch of things that real-life people have done in their real, depressed lives, to try to look after themselves a little bit and to introduce this whole 'self-care' malarkey to their otherwise dark and difficult days.

Maybe there'll be something in this list that seems achievable. Maybe you'll read it and then burn this book. Who's to say?

- 'When I'm having a really dark day, if I can muster it, I'll take a really hot bath and listen to music.'
- 'A pint of ice cream. Full fat. Eaten with a teaspoon.'
- 'Honestly this may be something very few relate to, but if I feel the beginnings of a dark cloud looming over me, I'll put on a film featuring Anna Faris (a personal favourite is *The House Bunny*). Something that doesn't challenge me or make me question aspects of my life I don't have the power to control will help ground me.'
- 'Puppies!'
- 'Stroking my dog. Getting out into sunshine (if I can make myself). Talking to friends (IRL, not social media).'
- 'Being spooned by my boyfriend. Helps every time.'
- 'I try to meditate on the worst days. It helps to blank the mind, if only for seconds.'
- 'I have a need to feel hugged all the time, so will put pressure on my body in some way to try to recreate that feeling.'
- 'I've started using the Headspace app and it's bloody brilliant. Most of my anxiety happens at night and it helps me to chill out.'
- 'Cuddles. Lots of cuddles.'

Just sleep on it, babes

Sleep is one of the most important things you can give yourself more of in an act of self-care. Getting enough good-quality sleep is life changing but sleep is both a gift and a tortuous minx. If it comes naturally it's a bloody delight; it's like dying. If you're asleep you escape everything else and can remain in oblivion and in darkness and without any consequence. If you can't sleep then you're in turmoil; everything is worse at night, from the inevitable death of everyone you love to that ominous leak in the bathroom. But sleep can be bulging with nightmares so terrifying and vivid that you come to dread a slumber altogether. Insomnia steals the relaxation from you and replaces it with unnecessary mind aerobics. Bitch.

There was a time when I would sleep straight through a day if I could. I would nap after work. Constantly at the weekends, and go to bed early so I could quickly dissolve into darkness. But then that gift of oblivion left, and sleep – or the lack of it – turned into something I then feared. Sleep didn't come. When it did come, it didn't last. When it broke I would wake slick with cold sweat and gripped by a thick elastic band of searing pain around my jaw and skull after relentlessly grinding my teeth. Sleep wouldn't come back. Even as I lay in bed, eyes closed and utterly exhausted, sleep eluded me.

'Have you tried using lamps and relaxing for a while before you try to go to sleep?' is a real question that a doctor asked me. Omg! A lamp! You mean I shouldn't be running around a floodlit room and shining torches directly into my eyes and wondering why I'm not switching off? NO SHIT, SHERLOCK. The same doctor told me to look into 'sleep hygiene', which – spoiler alert – is a twee term for 'common fucking sense'.

Who are these people sitting bolt upright in a room full of LED disco lights, scrolling through a beaming feed of access to all the world's knowledge in their palm, with the TV blaring death metal in the background while they're necking a pint of Red Bull, claiming that 'they just can't get to sleep!' Actually, there are loads of these people who are doing the rest of us actual sleep-deprived insomniac wasters a disservice by claiming lack of sleep when they're realistically doing nothing to encourage it.

Sure, you could have sleep apnoea or be a sleepwalker or have a complicated breathing condition or share a bed with someone who sleep-slaps you in the face every six minutes, but the sleep disruption and unpredictability that comes with depression really is something else.

Depression and sleep have a very Ross-and-Rachel style of relationship. Being depressed can make you need to sleep for seventeen hours a day and make you unable to pull your lead-like limbs out of bed for an entire (not so fragrant) week. Being depressed can also leave you lying wide awake at night while the rest of the country snores, and you're unable to get a wink of rest and your eyes are burning and your heart is racing and your gut is hollow and aching.

How can one illness have two such contradictory effects? I spoke to a psychiatry registrar, Dr Ken Adams, who told me that sleep and depression have pretty interesting links:

Many people with depression also have anxiety, and the negative cognitive biases that come with depression (negative thoughts about the self, the world and the future) lend themselves easily to rumination – an anxiety presentation.

Needing to sleep for days will come from a lack of energy, which is one of the core symptoms of depression. There may, I suspect, also be links to dysregulation in the hypothalamic-pituitary-adrenal axis.

Um, sorry, what?

Sure, we're all familiar with our hippocampus and its judging panel making 'executive decisions' for us, and how the depression demons just big fat swoop on in there and cause everything to shut down. But now, brain fans, we're onto a different part of our grey matter: the hypothalamus.

The hypothalamus is positioned towards the base of our brain and about the size of a 5p coin. Although teeny, it's super-important. Maybe a bit like Napoleon, or Kylie Minogue. The hypothalaminogue is essentially the teensy traffic controller, helping to regulate hormone release from our pituitary gland and generally quite interested in emotions, body temperature, appetite, sexual behaviour and the wily minx of sleep.

Serotonin helps regulate our sleep, and seeing as you're reading this joyful book of unbridled bliss, I'm gonna hazard a guess that your serotonin levels could also do with a re-stock, so I'll just move quickly on from that. Thanks, hypothalaminogue, for holding back on the good stuff.

Research has suggested that people with depression have a hypothalamus up to 5 per cent larger than people without, and that the severity of the depression can even directly correlate to the size of the hypothalamus.[32]

I went through a time of waking up at 3.42 a.m. every single night for what seemed like a year but was probably a couple of months. It was bizarre, like some kind of tragic, sad alarm clock injecting my chest with gas clouds of despair that woke me up as they billowed around the rest of my body, spreading a palpably painful toxicity through my veins. I would wake up with physical pain in my chest and a tyre-sized rock in my stomach, and lay awake crying silent, hot tears for hours.

I went through another time of having to call in sick to work because, well, it was 11.30 a.m. and I wasn't at work yet because I'd gone back to sleep. Not hungover, not with the flu, I went back to sleep and stayed asleep for the next eighteen hours. This happened every day for a week.

Then we're in some kind of blame-game again: do you sleep or wake because you're depressed, or are you depressed because your sleep is so messed up that your mind can't handle it any longer? Is it even possible to have a sleep disorder without being depressed? Is it possible to be depressed without your sleep being affected?

Perhaps more immediately pressing: how do you get to sleep when you're finding it impossible? Of course, different things will work for everybody and I'm not going to insult you with basic top tips like 'get to bed and read before you sleep' or 'no caffeine after 4 p.m.', but here are some other potential solutions I've gleaned from others:

- Listen to Stephen Fry narrating *Harry Potter*, even if you don't care for it.
- Recount all the exact things you did in the day and try to think of exactly what they were to the tiniest detail. Your mind will get bored and shut off.
- Concentrate on breathing and breathe all the way in for five seconds, and then all the way out for five seconds. Keep doing this until you sleep.
- Harry Styles on the Calm app (this sounds like it would keep me quite awake tbqh but at least you might get a saucy dream out of it if you do nod off).

- An audiobook of something you've already read, so you're not engaged but are relaxed instead.
- Listen to the soybean forecast. It's an actual thing and dull as hell.

There has been research into actually attempting to change sleep patterns as a treatment for depression. This is called triple chronotherapy and involves medical intervention in order to change your sleeping patterns. It's a system where, basically, your bedtime is changed to either be later or earlier. Triple chronotherapy 'is a combination of sleep deprivation, sleep phase advance and bright light therapy that has been shown to induce accelerated and sustained remissions in bipolar depression.'[33]

It's all about resetting your internal body clock – your circadian rhythm. Most of the treatments seem to begin with one night of no sleep whatsoever, until you've been awake for thirty-six hours and can go to bed at around 5 p.m. the next day. But then you get woken up at 1 a.m., stay awake until 7 p.m., are woken again at 3 a.m. and can't go to bed again until 9 p.m. Then on the last day you get woken up from your 9 p.m. sleep at 5 a.m, and you're off back to bed at 11 p.m.

Following a 7 a.m. wake-up call the next morning, you will have established a normal sleeping pattern and be on the road to recovery. Apparently.

A lot of bright-light therapy is used to help keep you awake, which is basically just surrounding you with some alarmingly bright lights, like the ones that are used to help treat seasonal affective disorder. OK, it actually involves you having to have a very bright light (about ten times brighter than your average household lightbulb) a foot away from you for thirty minutes as you go about your business reading the paper or having a snack thinking of death or however you spend your time.

Obviously, I'm just giving a summary here and not recommending any kind of wild sleep experimentation of your own – depression gives you enough of that already. But isn't it interesting that changing your sleep could be powerful enough to change your mental health?

(Yes.)

Upon a google I see that the only place in the UK that offers this treatment is the Priory, but I've written about it now so it's staying in the book.

Anyway, the Priory reckon that 'triple chronotherapy has been found to lead to a rapid response in up to 50 per cent of patients, resulting in significant improvements in their depression symptoms after only a few days. This response rate increases to two-thirds of patients after six months.'

There's a scientific reason that we often wake up feeling like we have more clarity or focus than we did the night before: sleep can actually clear our brain. If we're not sleeping well, we're not clearing our brains out, and are letting all the plaque and demons pile up and take over.

Also, as we snooze our lymphatic systems drain and filter neurotoxins in our bodies, taking them away from the brain. Alzheimer's sufferers have build-ups of plaques in their brains, which could prevent synapse functioning. Sleep, man. Sleep.

So really, the sleep weirdness and the self-loathing and the overly stressful/hormonal-feeling days are nothing to do with you just being a bit of a dick. There's a tiny pop star in your brain that's been given some extra-large spoons to dish out the hormones with, and on top of that, they can't read measurements so are well and truly messing you up. It's not your fault.

Self-care to try to combat self-hatred that mainly involves using the calendar on your phone:

- Note all your plans in your phone calendar, and take time to add in plans for yourself to take some time out when you can anticipate feeling crappy.
- Also, note how you're feeling in your calendar. This could be with an emoji or a word or whatever works for you, but having a clear, visual representation of your activities and your mood should present some patterns or links to you, so you can start to be more self-aware and thus on the road to self-care.
- If you can, note down what you did in the evenings if you didn't have any plans. This could be 'early night', 'sofa with wine', 'healthy dinner' or 'pizza' or 'bath' or anything, to see if there are ways you treat yourself that impact your mood positively or negatively.

Basically, become your own detective and investigate yourself. By now it's clear that you can't look after yourself until you've figured out what you need or what you're missing, or even what changes there could be to make. Trench coat and deerstalker optional.

The clapbacks

It's nice that someone's suggesting things to try to make you feel nice (#nice), but... no.

'That might work when you're sad, but I have clinical depression and a bit of lavender won't cure it.'

'Oh, I didn't realize you could get face masks for eternal gloom. Which ones do you use?'

'I do try to look after myself but it's hard when you don't care about yourself. What do you do to make yourself feel less crap?'

'Is there a bubble bath that removes internal darkness?'

CHAPTER 9

But you've got such an awesome job, dude

When a friend killed himself this past year, one of the most common reactions I heard was shock that he 'went through with it when he was just about to start such a cool new job', or concern along the lines of, 'Oh, was he not having a good time at work, then?'

Sure, a great job can put a spring in your step and give you a sense of purpose and satisfaction, and it can even inject you with some feelings of achievement if you find that you're actually quite good at something. But if you're depressed, completing a project will hardly dent the doom. If you're suicidal, you'll do it anyway. A job is not the only thing to live for.

Shamefully, I know I've definitely spat out a few 'Ah, come on, mate, at least have the weekend to sleep on it!'-themed comments when the London Underground has croaked to a halt after a devastatingly common train-track suicide on a Friday night. 'Why didn't they just quit their job if they hated it so much?' people ask, infuriated at the twenty-minute delay this person has added to their journey. 'Couldn't they have done it early on a Saturday?' wonder those who will have forgotten about this minor inconvenience within the next hour.

When that friend killed himself, it transpired that he devastatingly didn't ever make it to the office for the last day of his old job. 'Why didn't he hold on to see if things got better?' people asked.

Because, in his eyes, things won't get better, Linda. It's not about the job, it's about the black, syrupy tar of despair that's sludged around your brain and firmly stuck itself there, immovable by the brightest of days and the perkiest of colleagues. It's not about the job, it's about feeling like you are at the absolute darkest depths of the bottom of hell, and the way out is so steep and unclimbable that even a step towards the rock face is impossible. It's not about the job, it's about wishing that you had never been born. That you were never cruelly given this burden of life without ever asking for it, and now finding yourself wading through all-encompassing white-hot fire every day just to make it through.

The fact that 'Oh, man, their job must have been awful' even comes to mind is a reflection of how overworked we all are, and how much importance is placed on work compared to everything else that makes up a person's life.

It's never really about the job.

I think that by planning the date like that (we'll never know how long he planned it for, but 'they' do say that people who die by suicide plan the event far in advance, to be certain that they're prepared and that it won't fail), he was absolving himself of responsibilities. He planned that particular date to be sure that his suicide wouldn't inconvenience anybody at work because they needed to have that meeting with him about social media acquisition. He planned it to be sure that he didn't leave anyone with a burden of finishing something that he started, even with the very last thing he ever did.

But! That's not to say a job can't impact your mental health, of course. A job can mean everything as much as it can mean nothing. It's what you do nearly every day of your adult life, and if you have colleagues then you'll likely spend more time with them than you will with your family or partner. A bad job, or a job that you're bad *at*, can surround you in a pit of gloom and make you feel like any lights at the end of the tunnel have been unplugged. A boring job will make time drag and encourage you to dwell on what a failure you are, and an awful boss will make you feel worthless. Working night shifts or unsociable hours can leave you overtired and feeling lonely, and working in a huge office of people can be exhausting.

Working for yourself adds a whole different pile of pressure to your days, and working from home can be very isolating as well as blurring the lines between relaxation space and work space, and thus make us feel like we should be working all the time, as we'll all remember from the Covid lockdown.

When you're depressed, working from home can be very risky for both your employment status and your mental health. You're never too far from your bed and pyjamas, and submitting to life under the duvet cover is far more appealing than endless Zoom calls. Missing opportunities for social interactions isn't good for your brain, and for many people (me included, I shall reluctantly admit) having to be somewhere every day helps combat feelings of worthlessness. Although there are fewer distractions from colleagues and surprise meetings, it's a lot harder to have meaningful communications when you're not face-to-face.

When lockdown began it was a joy not to stuff myself onto

an underground train to commute to work, and to be able to get work done quickly without being 'borrowed for a bit'. The pressure of the office performance was off and the exhaustion from always being 'on' started to ebb away. But so did my motivation, and I soon found myself lapsing back into days spent in the darkness, drinking too much and not being kind to myself. When you only have to show up for yourself, you really won't bother if you don't think you're worth it.

So, how to manage it? For me, structure is helpful. Setting myself a lunch hour and getting outside for a walk during that time is invaluable, as is setting a stop-time for the end of the day, closing the laptop and leaving the house again. Even a short walk around a block gives me some separation, as it's easy to just continue working into the night when you've got nowhere else to be or nothing else to do. To keep being productive I split my tasks into lots of teeny ones, and write them down on a to-do list. This helps make the work seem achievable, and means you get way more of that satisfying cross-through of what you've accomplished. Another good tip for home-workers is to set up a designated work space that can be packed away or put out of sight when you're not working, rather than just working on the sofa. Having clear differences between your home space and your work space can take some of the pressure off.

Work can be all-consuming. Work is how we live. Hopefully we work to live and not live to work, as the saying goes, but when your work is the thing providing your quality of life then how can you not live to work? Work can so easily take over your life; we spend more time at work than we do out of work, generally, and our jobs hugely affect our sense of self-worth and validity. Having been at both burnout and boredom, I really don't know which is worse. When I was bored, I felt even more worthless than usual, my confidence was non-existent because I felt like I wasn't useful on a day-to-day basis, and all my friends had 'exciting work updates!!!!!' whereas I had... nothing.

When I was burnt out I still had all these feelings, but just didn't realize they were there underneath the stress and the pressure.

Sometimes I wish I was still going through burnout – or that I was at least on the edge of it. As I write this, I know I am doing a mediocre job at work, at best, because I just genuinely do not care. I don't care about anything. I don't care about making things 'the best month ever' or the 'most impactful video ever' or 'getting the most views ever'. I don't care about meeting my work 'goals' set by my boss, or if someone is coming in late every day. They're probably depressed, too – I'll cut them some slack.

This would be the same in any job, in my current state. I'm fully aware that I'm not working to my potential or impressing anyone, and I honestly do not care one single ounce. I can't care about anything, and fuck, I try. We already know that depression makes our brains struggle to make decisions or form future plans, and when you've pretty much given up on caring about your own life, what else can have any jeopardy?

I'm occupied but unenthused, and I believe truly that it would be the same even if I was employed as Cara Delevingne's personal cheek-kisser, as Shaggy's personal oil-rubber-inner-on-his-shoulders, or as Chief Puppy Stroker in a baby-animal farm.

Actually, I might have to think about the puppies.

But still, the majority of depressives will not kill themselves because of a shitty job and it is infuriating when the immediate response is to comment on how things 'must have been worse at work than we thought'. There are other things going on. Always.

I still can't figure out if the immediate response to suicide being about the person's job is a genuine lack of understanding of depression, or a lazy deferral tactic because this person actually understands depression all too well, and they want to brush something off as being all someone's boss's fault rather than admit that they, too, have felt close to the mark before. Surely it must be the latter? Surely everyone feels this way all the time? Surely nobody can *actually* think that someone wanted to end their life *just* because work is shit.

Let's face it (if you weren't bummed out enough by this work chat already then do brace yourself for some more Honest Doom): as millennials, work for us all is mostly fifty shades of crap.

We are way too aware of the fact that the majority of millennials entered the workforce when the workforce was actually collapsing on our approach because the Boomers had messed it all up for us with their mortgages and some *Wolf of Wall Street* stuff that I still don't entirely understand...

We all went out to find jobs in the time that those heinously smug '30 under 30' lists were created, when there were barely thirty available jobs in London, let alone smaller cities. For each of those thirty jobs there were 650 applicants, and for each of those 650 applicants about 400 were more qualified than we were because they'd just been made redundant from their decent job, so our only option was to intern for free and work in a pub afterwards for a sweaty six hours before we could finally relax with a refreshing, room-temperature WKD Blue.

Simpler times. WKD Blue? *Takes puff of cigarette.* I haven't had one of those in years.

So yeah, don't be even meaner to yourself for being a sucker for your job – it took you bloody long enough to find one in the first place, and if you've managed to get one that you were actually remotely excited to apply for then WELL DONE, LOVE.

But what happens when you're doing a job that you don't want to lose, but the gang of decision makers in your brain have had all the motivation sucked out of them by the demons and are thus not exactly helping you perform at your best?

It can be embarrassing to admit that you actually *do* care about what you do for a living, right? That you actually don't 'think you should be paid more for this shit' or that you were tricked into it under false pretences. It's FINE to like your job. It's GREAT! But it's not so great to make it the most important thing in your life, meaning more important than, you know, your sanity.

For a while I put way too much value on my job – I think everyone does in their twenties, right? As millennials we're surrounded by articles about the multi-millionaire CEOs who are 'only 23!!!!', just as we enter the declining job market with an increasingly competitive landscape. We largely joined the workforce at a time when the workforce was collapsing, and can easily feel trapped in a job because of a fairly severe lack of other options and extreme competition for anything that is actually available.

Of course, that means when we do get a job we actually like or even care about, we're bound to put pressure on ourselves to keep it, to be good at it and to not get replaced in favour of someone younger and cheaper. We pop out of school with a half-baked ambition (woah, remember ambition?) and set ourselves on a course to Get a Dream Job.

For me, the dream was to be working in magazines, and by Jove I got a job at one! Interviewing heroic teenage girls for *Sugar* magazine was incredible; from girls who'd escaped cults to girls who'd watched their mum run off with their boyfriend, it was such a varied and satisfying job (that paid the princely sum of £9k a year). Then there were the boybands, oh, the boybands.

One day my actual job was to *spray members of JLS with oil and then rub it around their torsos* so they looked sweaty for a shoot in a boxing ring. I still went home and cried and hoped not to wake up in the morning.

Another time a colleague and I got One Direction to see if they could all fit in the same giant pair of knickers together, for absolutely no reason other than it would make a fun video. I spoke to David Beckham about his hair, went on a plane with Rihanna for a week and waited in lavish hotel suites to interview Channing Tatum and Matthew McConaughey about their new male stripper film. It was the best, but I was still living the worst in my mind. Please, please don't feel like an ungrateful, entitled snowflake if you've got a job that's seemingly incredible, but you're still burning internally.

Trying to get through a day at work with your misery unnoticed is no easy feat, and personally I've always found myself acting up to such an extent that people actually sometimes thought I was 'a bit of a laugh' – which is laughable in itself really as I was simultaneously wondering if I died how long it would be before anyone would notice, and if it would mess up any projects we were working on in the office.

But let's be honest, talking to anyone about your depression can be a struggle, let alone your boss. I've written about depression for years and I *know* that in the long run it could be helpful for my manager to get full disclosure, but I very much subscribe to the school of keeping it to yourself for as long as possible. I figure if it's not actually impacting my work then there's no need to bring it up, and that when it actually makes its way out of my brain and into the office then, *then* I'll bring it up.

It's literally your manager's job to manage your workload, though, and make sure that you're not being overwhelmed or left bored. It does make sense for your boss to be aware of your mental health struggles so that they can support you when you need it, but I get it. You might not need support at work because you're so good at faking it.

It's tricky as a manager, too, when I can see signs of depression in employees but they so clearly do not want to talk about it. I was once managing a girl who had started coming into the office gradually later and later, and looking more and more sombre every day. As a boss, I can ask her if she's OK and what support or flexibility she needs from me to be able to do her job properly. I have to respect her privacy, but I tell her that if there's anything that's affecting her work then we can find a way to work around it together. Whether that's working from home, a more flexible schedule or taking time off altogether. I can see the sadness in her eyes, the slowness in her gait and the exhalations of defeat in her posture.

'I'm fine,' she says. 'I won't be late again. There aren't any changes we can make, it's OK.'

So that's that. I can't force her into telling me anything she doesn't want to, and if she says there's nothing affecting her ability to be able to do her job properly then I have to assume she's just slacking off and being lazy and entitled, right? If she doesn't tell me she's depressed then I can't do anything to help her.

It's nobody's obligation to tell anyone about their depression, but I would encourage you to say something to a trusted manager if it's getting to the stage where your depression is affecting your work. Usually, I'm (as I'm sure you can imagine) a stoic, professional businesswoman in the office, but sometimes the demons aren't hidden behind walls of tasks and to-do lists and P&Ls and politics and other office crap to keep them away. Sometimes they get out and mess everything up, and sometimes I have to abruptly leave the office because I can't stop crying, and desk-sobbing isn't really a great look.

If I'm going to need to do this every now and again, my manager needs to know why. Otherwise I am just an unreliable employee bunking off work or 'mysteriously getting sick', which looks a lot like a fake-out.

From a manager's perspective, I want to know what's affecting anyone who's working with me and what I can do to support them. If it's a mental illness – or any illness or situation that I might not understand – I need someone to be as specific as possible when they tell me what's happening with them. Do they have anxiety and need to leave the office for a quick walk every hour because they panic in small spaces? Do they have OCD and thus a terrible time leaving the house in the morning and will probably be late a lot?

If someone said, 'Just to let you know, I have depression. It's not affecting my work, but I'll let you know if it feels like it is or might,' then that would be a start. But alas, we'd both need to have an idea of how it might affect the work, which can be tricky to pre-empt with something like depression and the surprise ways it decides to mess up your life. A pretty good standard of informing a manager could be something like: 'I want to do a good job here but to do that I'm going to need to be able to work around my depression, so it's important that you understand that I have it. It doesn't affect my work every day, but when it does I'll let you know, and will likely need some flexibility around working from home when I'm feeling really low, as it's not professional of me to bring that state of mind into the office and to my colleagues.'

But what about if you don't work in a typical office environment, or you can't work from home? What about if you already work from home and your depression means you're always doing the 'at home' bit but never the 'working' bit? It can be a lot trickier when you're obliged to stay at your workplace to do the work, or when going home means that you don't get paid.

Here are some tips from people who do this, and how they cope:

- 'I take advantage of flexible hours and try to work when the fewest number of people are in the office, and leave early for afternoon naps. Then there are days when I need to work at home so I can cry freely.'
- 'In the morning I do a mindfulness or meditation practice. On my commute, I listen to a motivational/self-development audiobook. At lunch, I take a walk and get some air.'
- 'I walk home at the end of every work day because I need the space. Then when I'm at home I need a big hug.'
- 'I'm a teacher, so I get through one lesson at a time and focus on the children rather than myself, which works. Plus, the persona I adopt for teaching detaches me from the depression totally (which has always made me wonder).'
- 'I live close by yet I drive to work – that way if ever I am really upset or exhausted, I know I have a safe place I can retreat to. I always bring my headphones to work in case I need to listen to some peaceful music to distract my

thoughts. I also have a SAD lamp – I'm not really sure if it's just a placebo effect but I find it can lift my spirits anyway.'

- 'I get through the day at work fine, it all comes to a head when I'm home and it's quiet. I take long shower after long shower.'

- 'I seem to have the opposite of claustrophobia and always find comfort in a small space where I feel compressed. I'll go and sit in a very small space, or literally sit under my desk.'

- 'I make sure I take time for a nice cup of tea and some chocolate, and a quick walk in the fresh air in the afternoon.'

But then there are those of us whose jobs have actual real meaning beyond oiling up boybands (meaningful as that is, of course) and who can't just nip out for some air if they're feeling wobbly, because they're in the middle of brain surgery or teaching a class. There are people whose job it is to save lives, to care for the vulnerable or sick, or to decide who is guilty in court. There are people who have to drive ambulances skilfully enough to reach someone before it's too late. There are people who take on the educating and personal problems of six classes of thirty ten-year-olds. There are people whose jobs are so crucial to society that, whooooof, I can't even imagine how it would feel to be depressed at work, feeling like you're idiotically focusing on your own cranky brain when there are lives or minds very much at stake and very much in your hands. HOW do you deal with depression when if you take time for yourself, someone might die?

To help me answer this, I spoke to a gal named Emma who has worked as a nurse for fourteen years and been on the front-line of some major events both in the UK and in Afghanistan. She suffers from anxiety and PTSD as a result of her work, and her story is both affecting and typical of people suffering mental health problems in countries where the health service is strained. I chose to share it in the hopes that others who've been passed around from waiting list to waiting list will feel less alone, seeing as there's not much I can do about the actual waiting lists themselves.

Emma strives to support all her patients and colleagues as much as she can through her twelve-hour shifts, but it often comes at the detriment of herself and her own wellbeing. She told me:

> It's taken me a long time to figure out how best to manage these situations, and in particular when needing to take a break. The nurses can't all take their breaks at the same time. It can become overwhelming and stifling, with no headspace or ability to take a five-minute time-out.

Emma's passion to help people and work in a challenging environment came to a peak in 2012 when she was deployed to Afghanistan as a civilian nurse. As with most people's 'dream job', once you actually get to them you realize it's quite terrifying. As a nurse on the frontline of a war zone, it was traumatizing.

Upon Emma's return to the UK she found herself struggling with readjustment and anxiety, and participated in some CBT sessions to try to help her work through it. She felt the work was done after about four sessions, though, and dropped out as she was paranoid about wasting the time of fellow health professionals. On reflection, she says, this was a poor decision, and her PTSD caught up with her after being exposed to traumatic amputations in the field.

Emma describes the memories as vividly detailed and distressing, and they came to her in flashbacks most days. As she was continuing to work in a major trauma centre, she was also living with the fear that a similar patient would be brought into her hospital and she would have to relive her horror once again:

It was like a wrecking ball of fear as soon as I made the journey into work and I developed palpitations the moment I stepped through the door. I felt exhausted from the anxiety, which had a knock-on effect on my concentration, memory and ability to sleep. I had little capacity to process anything. But as I was often the most senior nurse on shift, I had to maintain a sense of 'keep calm and carry on', even though I was starting to crumble underneath.

A psychologist suggested that I would benefit from EMDR (eye movement desensitization and reprocessing) and pointed me in the direction of self-referral to my local borough's psychology services. After a lengthy telephone consultation, I was told my symptoms were only mild and there was a ten–twelve-month waiting list for individualized support, with no availability for group sessions for at least another two–three months.

I was also told about private therapy, but the only options for EMDR were completely unaffordable for me (we are talking up to £120 per session, with a minimum recommendation of six sessions). I had tried mindfulness apps but they weren't helpful when trying to combat anxiety on the busy and often noisy commute to work.

I was reliving the pain every single time I had to explain my mind, only for someone to turn around and tell me that my symptoms were considered mild. For the very fact that I didn't say I was suicidal, I was deemed to have a minor problem.

Was that my next option? To create a lie and say the worst things, just in a desperate plea for someone to listen? I couldn't bring myself to do it.

Emma eventually, after four months, had an appointment arranged to see a psychologist. She also moved out of London, which has made a marked difference to her health and happiness:

Living away from the city and closer to the ocean, for me, has played a significant part in improving my overall wellbeing. It still worries me that I may face the same problems down the line, and as I say this, it still baffles me as to how difficult, painful and obstructive that whole experience was.

I only hope that there will be better access to mental health resources and more understanding for nurses/allied health professionals in the future, as we will all need it.

We know that the depression demons don't care about the roof over your head, your loving family, your friends or your amazing job. Even people who have significant, incredible jobs where they save lives (not that my roles as 'digital content strategist' are insignificant… ahem) aren't immune.

My magnificent sister happens to be a doctor (I say 'happens', it was very much on purpose following years of intensive study and exams), and whenever I find myself wanging on about something trivial that happened to me in my office I always feel like I should live in the Box of Shame for even *thinking* about *telling* her about my work crap, when her 'work crap' is literally life or death.

'You can't keep apologizing for not being a doctor,' she tells me. 'Everyone's daily stresses are relative. Just because you're not a doctor doesn't mean you can't have had an awful day.' She's so wise. This is why she's a doctor.

Doctors, accountants, farmers, administrators, chefs, waitresses, gardeners, circus clowns... you name it, it seems like this 'competitive busyness' is pushing us all to the brink. The world has less money and is generally getting fewer people to do more work for a cheaper price. Our inbuilt fear of losing everything makes us push ourselves harder, and it's not surprising we're all burning out.

We check emails when we escape to the loo at a house party or when we're out for dinner. We open our inboxes when we're in bed next to someone we could be having sex with, but instead we're both staring at screens and worrying that we haven't responded to the emails sent to us at absurd times outside our working hours, because everyone else at work seems to have replied immediately. We have our jobs in our hands twenty-four hours a day, and as we press snooze on our alarm clocks we're greeted with notifications about new crises to solve and tasks to complete.

Don't even START on the work-based WhatsApp groups that have popped up now. So now people have a direct line of communication into your hand that you will always see, no matter what time it is or day it is or holiday you're on. It's much easier to block out time to both check emails and to keep out of your inbox than it is to plan your WhatsApp messaging.

This is hardly an alien concept; we've been socially conditioned to think that we should be working all the time. We should always be 'on', we should be grinding the grind hard and if we're not doing the actual work then we should always be looking for networking opportunities.

We're worried about losing the work we do have and masking it by sending our friends memes about arriving at work two hours late but with an iced coffee and a blow dry. We work when we're not *at* work, and cover it up with emails to our work pals telling them how we're 'sooo done with this shit!' but actually, we're kind of addicted. We've put Instagram filters on our real life to hide that we're burning out underneath them.

Millennials aren't lazy, we're workaholics.

But getting through a work day when the depression demons are having a lovely swim around your brain… that's a tough one. If you've already used up all your holiday allowance to stay in bed with your demons, there are a few things that might help you get your work done when you're feeling like death.

- **Make lists.** Break every task down into smaller parts so they don't seem too monstrous. Crossing through each point when you're done should give you a sense of accomplishment, no matter how small.
- **Take lots of notes.** Your memory is probably total crap if you're feeling really dark, and you won't be able to recall conversations or instructions as well as usual. If you can't

take notes, you could take a recording or ask the person speaking to follow up with an email.

- **Have breaks.** Whether it's stepping outside for some air, going to cry in the pub loos across the road or just going to say hi to a colleague, change it up.
- **Breathe.** OK, this one sounds a bit daft, but take a really slow, deep breath inwards until you feel like you can't fit any more air inside you. Hold it for three seconds, then breathe it all out really, really slowly, until you feel empty. It can help calm the demons a little.

Remember it's illegal to be discriminated against at work because of a health condition, and that having good mental health will make you do your job better. If there's no way on earth you would ever dream of telling your boss about it, try telling a colleague who you trust. Asking for a quick chat somewhere private and quiet is a good idea, before explaining to them that while it might have seemed as though you're totally off your game recently and are becoming a bit bone idle, you're actually depressed and struggling with productivity and motivation at the moment. The instant response from them might be to wonder why you're telling them, so if there's anything that you need from them then now's the time to say it. 'Do you think you could spare a few minutes to look over XYZ/go for a quick walk around the block in the afternoons/help me make a to-do list' – or if you don't need anything from them, tell them that, too. At the very least, when you're having particularly dark days it's helpful to have someone else look over your emails or work before you send it out – depression can really quickly remove all kindness and niceties from your vocabulary.

Also, let's keep playing the lottery just in case we can become gazillionaires and never have to go to work again.

The clapbacks

What to say when someone insists you can't possibly be depressed because you've got SUCH a good job, I mean just LOOK at your CV, it's BRILLIANT, don't be sad. You've got it made!

'Oh, you're right! I forgot that people who do statistical analysis and data configuration can't be depressed.'

'So did Robin Williams.'

'I do have a good job, but it's not the only thing to live for. I wish having a great job like mine would help my illness go away, but it doesn't.'

'That's true. I can't imagine how shit you must feel with your job, then.'

CHAPTER 10

You're always so FUN though, pal

OH, SORRY I DIDN'T BRING MY RAINCLOUD ON A STRING TO HANG OVER ME.

Ahem. You know that thing where you need to pee a little bit, and then as soon as you get home and put your key in the front door you feel like the pee has taken over your body and you're just gonna explode with the force of it all if you can't go RIGHT ACTUAL NOW? Well, that, but with crying.

A lot of this seems to be about crying, but honestly, living with this is a lot about crying. Sometimes I cry so much that I feel like I might choke on my own saliva, and then I hope desperately that I do. Sometimes I cry so much I vomit. Sometimes I cry so much that I can't stop and I have to *make myself vomit* to see if it helps, as the heaving and the burning and the wrenching and the coughing feels like a purge, like I might be getting the blackness out of me. If it doesn't leave me, then at least I've punished myself for being such a disappointment. Why the fuck am I so miserable, me, with all my limbs and immediate family still intact? What do I have to be upset about? Get a grip, love.

A lot of the funniest people are often – and I must stress that often does not mean *always* – depressed. There is pain behind laughter, which can commonly come from a place of darkness. Look at Robin Williams. 'What did he have to be sad about?' asked morons in droves after his 2014 suicide. 'But he was so funny, you wouldn't think he'd take his own life.'

There's a link between humour and depression, and it's no laughing matter. If you're feeling desperate inside, and entirely ashamed of the misery that burns, what better way to cover it up than by being funny?

Humour is a defence mechanism and can provide an impenetrable wall between the comic and their crowd; if they're always funny and making people smile, then *they* must be smiling all the time, surely? They must have a BALL. Their life must be a RIOT. They must not be able to MOVE without making a joke. Hahahahahahaahahahahahahahaahahahahahahaha no.

Chris Rock called comedy 'blues for people who can't sing', and Robin Williams, unsurprisingly, summed it up perfectly: 'I think the saddest people always try their hardest to make people happy because they know what it's like to feel absolutely worthless and they don't want anyone else to feel like that.'

At the time of writing, there are nine classifications of depression defined by psychiatric associations,[34] but 'laughing on the outside and dying on the inside' hasn't made it to the list just yet. I mean, depression is so different with every bugger carrying it around that there are certainly hundreds more distinctions of it that have yet to make it to any kind of official list, but I've personally found that reaching for the comedic angle can (if the joke lands, at least) make you momentarily not think about wanting to be dead.

Grasping for a punchline is well known as a defence mechanism;

a lot of people make jokes when they're uncomfortable or when they're trying to avoid talking about something intimate or painful. Humour helps us deal with a whole gaggle of horrible situations, and patients in severe emotional shock have been well documented as bursting out into uncontrollable fits of laughter as they try to process devastating news. Defence mechanism, sure. *Coping* mechanism? Most definitely.

Laughter releases positive chemicals. Dopamine and endorphins are so craved in a brain space that's severely lacking in serotonin, and laughter can give us a quick fix. Even when something trivially upsetting happens and we give ourselves a slap on the thigh and say, 'Oh well, you've gotta laugh, haven't ya!' we are explicitly directing ourselves to cover up pain with a bit of forced comedy. To make light or fun of a situation also makes us feel like we have some sort of control over it[35] – much like, say, if someone were to write a book about depression and litter it with crappy jokes. Shrug.

Personally, making other people laugh also makes me feel like I'm doing something to help someone else not feel as miserable as I feel all the time. It's the same false thought pattern that we talked about before: 'If they're laughing, they must be happy! I have saved someone from feeling pain. Please don't feel pain, other person over there, for I know what pain is and I want to keep you from it.'

It's been proven that experiencing low moods increases our capacity for empathy when we see others going through pain.[36] By experiencing darkness ourselves, we know what it's like to be trying to wade through the gloom, and spoiler – it's The Worst. With empathy comes 'empathic distress', when what little there is left of our heart breaks to see or consider someone else feeling even a tiny bit near as bleak as we've felt.

Empathy is a great quality to have; it helps you create close connections with people, and helps you forgive. It also makes you more anxious and can foster guilt in the empathizer; some scholars have noted that this could contribute to the huge amount of guilt that usually comes with depression.[37] Fun!

Despite all my wanging on about speaking up about mental health, there is still a stigma, and it might not be the first thing you want to talk about when you start a new job, for example, or meet new people. Enter: comedy! Humour can seem like the best cover-up for internal darkness – laughing people can't be depressed, right?! Wrong. Obviously, wrong.

Other studies have shown that people suffering from 'mood disorders' actually have functional and structural neural changes in the brain's neural circuit, right smack in the bits which affect empathic responses.[38] This means that depressed people (hollaaa!) can often have a surplus of empathy. This is depression fucking with your brain chemistry yet again, and is also a reason why so many of us who are depressed often feel like we're the ones to blame for the pain of others. Yep, as well as making you fill up with misery, depression also has a way of making you remarkably self-centred – even if the self-centring you're doing is putting yourself at fault for everything.

Of course, all this chatter about laughter and empathy is easy when you're out of the really thick quicksand. Depression in its rawest form removes the ability to produce any emotions apart from numbness. It sucks out all happiness or even false, plastic happiness, and empathy is a luxury that sounds foreign. Anyone else is unreachable, and any of life's other problems seem insignificant to the hollow pain of wanting everything to stop. The more I write about this particular pain of not wanting to live, the more I feel that someone reading it (hello? Is anyone reading it?) might think, 'Well, just go ahead and kill yourself then if the pain is *that* bad!' and of course THAT THOUGHT HAS CROPPED UP A BIT, HUN.

Sometimes the pain is so pure that it burns out of you in a silent, white-hot scream. It can't be visible because it's too hot. It can't be audible because it's too intense. You buckle and twist underneath it as it scalds from your chest out of your throat and all you feel is fire underneath the soaking layers of sweat and tears, and you wonder how you could die in this moment. What could you do to die right now? How could you end it? What the fuck are you brave enough to do that would put a stop to this and put you out of your misery and quiet your brain and give everyone else a relief?

Nothing.

Nothing, because you feel like a weak, writhing mess, twisting in sopping sheets and crying burning, silent tears. Nothing because you, too, feel nothing, and you're too scared to try to overdose in case it goes wrong and you end up a vegetable. You're too scared to use a knife in case you can't see it through and you become a 'cry for help'. You're too scared to do anything in case it doesn't work because you're too fucking weak, and then you end up living an even more pathetic and watched life, in the care of others who are trying to deprive you of the one thing you crave the most: oblivion. You're too scared to die, really, and just want the pain to stop. Living without the pain seems unimaginable. It burns.

My sadness is physical. It starts in my chest, a low thrum of despair that slowly gets louder, harder, as if my heart is pulsing dark sadness around my veins. Truly, I can feel it. It spreads down to my arms and into my fingers in a way that makes them ache and really physically hurt, while my chest feels heavy and my eyes are leaking and in an iron-clad scrunch. Maybe I'll get Botox when I'm happy.

A moment for the magic of faking everything through text messages. When you want to shut yourself away, sometimes all you need to do is turn your phone off. It's the only way people can get to you anymore, and it's highly unlikely that a friend will pop round unannounced to see if you're OK – this isn't *Gilmore Girls*. When you do decide to enter back into the world of connectivity, all you have to do is include a smiley emoji with your messages and everything will seem rosy to a recipient. I couldn't even begin to try to count how many messages with an overly smiley face I've sent to people while I've been sobbing at a pace that leaves me gagging on my own breath. So #blessed and #grateful for WhatsApp GIF responses.

This isn't to say that every funny person is dying on the inside and that anyone you know who's ever made you laugh is brimming over with self-loathing, but it's worth taking a moment for your mates who are so constantly side-splitting that they couldn't possibly be splitting inside. If, when you're alone with someone, they still turn things into jokes and reach for the punchline wherever possible, it's likely that they're not comfortable letting down their guard and showing you who they really are.

I'm not saying you should tell your mate that you're sick to the back teeth of their jokes and you just want to know what makes them miserable, but it's worth checking in and asking about the less comedic parts of their life. If things are glossed over with a stand-up routine, a 'that sounds hard, though, how do you actually feel?' is your bone to throw, letting them know that you're around if they ever want to drop the laughter track and talk.

Mostly, comedy is funny because it's sharply pointing out a very truthful observation that we all otherwise try to gloss over, and I guess that's what I'm trying to do here; point out the true awfulness of what depression can do to you, while poking fun at it along the way because, hey, if we've managed not to kill ourselves thus far, we might as well laugh about it. Making people laugh is an addictive experience and makes you feel a connection to others, whereas depression spends most of the time making you feel otherwise totally isolated.

Our brain's frontal lobe is host to the prefrontal cortex's control centre, which decides how we emotionally respond to things, and thus, if a joke is funny or not. If our panel of brain judges determines that, yes, that was quite a good joke Linda made and, yes, it's tickled us to laughter, the frontal lobe lights up and becomes very busy, sending a response to its pals in the occipital lobe (in the back of the brain) and down to our motor functions, meaning that we could slap a thigh or lean forward or generally have any physical response to good ol' Linda. Depression is temporarily taken over by Christmas lights of dopamine and serotonin and, fleetingly, doesn't stand a chance.[39]

Laughter is a gorgeous reaction to find yourself having to just about anything. I don't want to say that laughter is a privilege (because hell, we all feel guilty enough about our privileges) but there's of course a very deep end of the depression pool where laughter, or even the thought of being vaguely amused by anything ever again, is impossible. To laugh means that your frontal lobes are healthy enough to process humour (very different from the laughter you may involuntarily emit when being tickled, for example). The brains of depressed people show that the action in the frontal lobe is waaaay less than an 'average brain', and thus we struggle to respond with laughter or appreciate humour. In a depressed brain, the judges haven't bothered to turn up for joke-rating work, and the panel desks are left empty.

When I was in this particular funfair of depression, it was similar, I think, to a feeling of grief; feeling anxious and helpless alongside a deep sadness – perhaps for the loss of my former self, or for the hopelessness of what looks like a truly bleak and often pointless future. It's the constant simmering of thick, heavy tar just underneath your top layer of skin that boils over when you least need it to or are least expecting it to. It's a fog. It's a blindness. It's heavy limbs and a hollow chest, and wondering how you'll ever get through anything ever again.

When you're grieving, it's difficult to find a way to focus on anything. You become forgetful, and ignore your personal responsibilities (like washing or combing your hair). Your muscles weigh you down. Your sleep is sporadic. You can't pull the sadness from the front of your mind, and when you try to yank it away it just seems to wrap itself around the rest of your body instead, and you ache.

Comedy is not the same thing as happiness.

The thing is, nobody teaches us how to be sad. We're always taught that being happy is the only option, so we've become masters of faking it. I recently moved into a new rental apartment and even the fucking PLATES say 'Smile and be happy!' on them. Obviously they're all now smashed. Fuck you, sad-shaming chinaware.

Similarly to how being taught to do a self-assessment tax return might be more helpful than learning the theorem of Pythagoras, learning about the human brain and our emotions might be more helpful than, say, er, not learning about them. Emotional intelligence is (I reckon) one of the most admirable and worthwhile qualities a person can have, and unfortunately it usually comes after having significant lows and learning from them (and the ol' depression = empathy situation we just lolled our way through).

Imagine how different the world would be if we were taught how to feel feelings. If sadness and anxiety were ingrained in everyone as the totally normal feelings that they are, and not a sign of weakness or failure.

Imagine a world (sorry for sounding like a film trailer) where we allowed ourselves to feel our feelings, and never hid them or told ourselves to just get a grip. Would it be a tear-ridden, sobbing-in-the-streets planet of trust-falls and chanting circles? Or would everyone be kinder to one another, tell more jokes, make more effort to understand each other and suffer less at the hands of a patriarchy built on toxic notions that men should never show an emotional response unless it's anger or 'Let's go to CrossFit'?

Even when people tell me, Queen of Doom, that they're feeling low, my first response is an immediate need to make them feel better, and a phrase like 'Don't worry, it'll pass' is usually on the tip of my tongue because society has taught us to gloss over the gloom because 'it will get better'. But sometimes it doesn't, and if you've managed not to kill yourself (applause) then humour and over-the-top joviality is an absolutely acceptable mask, tonic and coping mechanism.

It's the whole 'sad clown paradox', where clowns and comedians create their humour out of deep pain, and use comedy as a way of releasing tension. It's using light-hearted humour when you're feeling tense and actually ripping up inside. It's Chandler from *Friends*. It's me! It's probably you, too, and dammit, honey, you tell those jokes if you need to.

But what if you do need to, and you can't? Depression isn't exactly known for feeling like a light tickle.

- If you can, then watching films, reading books and looking at social media accounts that talk honestly about mental health really helps it to feel more 'normalized', and the more you feel this, the closer you'll be to being able to joke about it. Instagram accounts that post 'depression memes' are controversial but personally, I find them hilariously relatable.
- Stand-up comedians often source their comedy from a pretty dark place. Their self-deprecating humour may well have a few relatable anecdotes and it's worth shoving on Netflix to see if you feel something.
- Focus on cheering up someone else. Sending a joke or a meme or a 'remember when we...' to someone you love will feel good, and hopefully put you in a more cheerful place even if just momentarily.

The clapbacks

Alrighty. So a shocked acquaintance is exclaiming how you can't possibly be depressed because 'you're always so fun', and perhaps suggesting that 'maybe you just feel a bit down'. What do you say to that? I'm gonna try some of these:

'Why, yes, I cover my pain with crappy jokes so that I don't cry or collapse in front of you. Now, an Irishman walks into a bar…'

'You're seeing my highlights reel. The rest of the film is a lot darker, and I like to just show the fun bits to my adoring public.'

'Honestly, I try to keep it light because inside it's so heavy, and we could all do with a bit more laughter.'

'Well, everyone thought Jimmy Savile was a charmer.'

CHAPTER 11

Maybe you should eat better, poppet

Some people (me) say that the true way to a person's soul is through the stomach. Some other people (twats) tell you to 'fast for a few days to detox the body and then you'll feel loads better'.

The thing with depression is that sometimes you fast for a few days unintentionally anyway, as it has a very peculiar effect on the appetite. Other times you find yourself reaching for a pint of ice cream, but instead realize you're living in a sub-par *Bridget Jones* cliché and it's gone straight to DVD. Other times, you feel like your sense of smell and taste have gone, and you eat things just to sort of… try and… feel something? The stronger the flavour the better. You're not actually hungry, just trying to get a reaction out of yourself. It's all very weird.

Annoyingly, there is a lot of research to prove that what we put in our mouths (steady on) has a direct relation not only to our physical health, but our mental health, too. As our messed-up brains consume over half of the nutrition and oxygen we get, this goes much further than 'I feel ashamed after eating another Domino's' or 'I feel really fantastic when I've had a KitKat Chunky'.

A fun study showed that when a sample of 152 depressed adults lived off a Mediterranean diet (high in vegetables, fruits, legumes, nuts, beans, cereals, grains, fish and olive oil) supplemented with fish oil, it led to a significant reduction in depression among the participants, which was then sustained for up to six months after the experiment.[40] What I'm saying – and what science is clearly saying – is to pack up your life and move to Spain immediately.

Of course, it's possible to eat like you're in an Olivio advert every day of your life and still be depressed (might as well crack into that Häagen-Dazs, hey?), but as with everything else, we're not all made equally and we'll all have different balances of body chemistry that make us need different things. The relationship between food and mental health is a complex one without one singular answer that will work for everyone – and that's before we even pop the cork of your wine stash and talk about the booze.

Food can be many things: it can be both a pleasure and an enemy, a thrill and a threat. It can be fuel for your engine, comfort for your soul and a way of self-medicating. It's also often the focal point of social activity.

There's been so much research about the impact food has on our mental wellbeing that it'd be silly to ignore it if you're struggling and have exhausted so many other avenues. Annoyingly, this particular area of research has been given an agonizingly New Age name: nutritional psychiatry. Moods 'n' foods would've been much better.

I've always been of the opinion that fasting to 'reset yourself' is as effective as going to the top of a high building to immediately overcome your crippling fear of heights; it ain't gonna work, honey. I can definitely subscribe to the school of giving yourself the best fuel for your optimum performance, as if we were all sports cars – but sports cars can't win races on fumes.

Fasting therapy is now 'a thing'. There's a 'fasting sanitorium' in Siberia (the actual place, not the 'social Siberia' we all know and love), which claims that willingly depriving yourself of all food and drink apart from water will leave you feeling energetic and refreshed. A similar clinic in Germany says that you should definitely experience its fasting services if you're suffering from depression, chronic fatigue or burnout, or if you are 'not quite healthy but not quite ill'.

The 'therapeutic centres' do say that you will be thoroughly examined by a doctor, and that if you are underweight, weak or 'emotionally or physically exhausted' you will be given supplements. Hmm.

Is this just a commercial ploy to get people to pay for no food?

Dr Giuseppe Aragona spoke to me about the alleged benefits of fasting, in between his work as a GP and for the online medical service Prescription Doctor.

'There is no medical research that assumes that fasting can "reset the mind" or "help the body" to detox,' he told me. Ha! 'In fact, quite the opposite. Fasting could lead to an increase in the amount of toxins circulating in the body due to an overworked liver and kidneys. Long-term fasting could lead to potential irreversible damage.

'Total fasting is widely demonstrated to be dangerous.'

Dr Aragona would advise against it, medically speaking (and, as a hungry, hangry, cranky, sad person with no medical qualifications whatsoever, I would tend to agree):

Claims that fasting may be healthy are, medically speaking, not true. Our bodies need an energy supply in its routine so that our brains can burn its favourite fuel (sugar) regularly.

A lack of sugar can lead our brains to malfunction (not in a judicial sense but a difficulty in making any kind of decision or leading to a lack of concentration) and lead our body to use alternative 'fuels' to work (like proteins, taken from our muscles or ketonic acids, that produce dangerous metabolites).

As we already know, because we've chatted a lot about how the brain functions in our depressive states, our brain's decision-making abilities and concentration centres are already pretty messed up because of our shoddy mental health. If depriving our sweet judging panel of key nutrients will make those functions even worse, then I (again, no medical qualifications) would advise everyone to go have a snack right now.

But if, for some reason, fasting is still appealing to you, there is a medically recommended way to approach it. Dr Aragona says:

If you are still interested in fasting, the safest way to achieve this would be a fasting mimicking diet (FMD). An Italian-American biogerontologist, Valter Longo, developed the fasting mimicking diet, which is a low-calorie, low-protein, low-carbohydrate, high-fat meal programme.

This programme is claimed to mimic the effects of periodic fasting or water fasting over the course of five days, while still

*aiming to provide the body with the nutrition it needs. FMD
is considered a periodic fast and it is proved to be effective.*

You tell me how that goes while I eat chips.

As we know, it's Instagram's world and we're merely existing in it, and social media is packed full of people who promote the benefits not of eliminating food altogether, but of drastically changing your food intake to a strict plant-based diet, after they did the same and claimed it cured their various illnesses and muscle aches.

The most famous is probably Ella Mills, socially known as @DeliciouslyElla, who, long story short, was suffering from postural orthostatic tachycardia syndrome (PoTS) in 2011 when she decided to try a diet change to ease her symptoms. PoTS sounds nasty; sufferers typically get a big dose of chronic fatigue, uncontrollable heart rates and palpitations, dizziness and a high risk of fainting, shaking and sweating, headaches, trouble sleeping, chest pain and 'brain fog' – problems with concentration, memory and thinking in general. Huh, sounds a lot like the symphony of shit that comes hand-in-hand with depression, doesn't it?

In the interests of 'I'll try anything to feel better as long as I don't have to stop eating', I thought it worth digging into this a bit more. Ella found that her symptoms were pretty much completely alleviated after giving up gluten, meat, sugar and dairy... but it took two years. This sounds pretty limiting, but luckily we live in the future and there are countless substitutes as well as natural options available if we wanted to try to follow this path.

Um, it doesn't sound fun, though. I'm sad enough already without saying goodbye to my cheese on toast.

Food and emotions are so tightly bound together that it's difficult to even think about making such a drastic change – and personally, I don't bloody want to. There is a whole genre of food called comfort food for a very good reason. Tastes and smells of food can remind us of happier or more simple times, times when we were being looked after or times when we had less misery. Also, sometimes Alphabetti spaghetti just really makes you feel taken care of.

My favourite remedy of reaching for a pint of ice cream when I'm sad usually provides me with a small amount of relief. I could write a separate book on the emotional benefits of ice cream alone. It helps comfort misery, it aids a desperate hangover, it's perfect when you're stoned and tastes like perfection when eaten outside, from a cone, on a sharply cold day.

Look, there was even a study that scientifically proved that eating ice cream in the morning stimulates your brain and increases mental activity.[41] Researchers studied the abilities of two groups of people when performing tasks in the morning. One group was given ice cream immediately on waking, the other group wasn't. Lo and behold, the ice-cream group performed better than the group for whom Ben & Jerry were a distant memory.

'But it's probably just the cold!' said the naysayers. 'Cold will wake up the brain! It doesn't have to be ice cream!' they spat out with their potent anti-joy-venom (I imagine). 'OK,' the researchers said, 'we'll try something else.' So the same experiment was completed but this time ice-cold water was given in place of the ice cream. The cold-water participants still performed better at the tasks than the group without any cold morning stimulant, but – and I cannot stress this enough – **they didn't perform as well as the test group who had the ice cream.**

Yes, this is vague, but it also vaguely says ice cream is a health food, so let's go with it.

There was another study that showed ice cream 'lights up the happy parts of the brain' but the researchers didn't supply much supporting evidence, and the study was implemented by Unilever – who own Carte D'Or – so I'm suspicious.

Anyway. Other researchers looked at how fatty foods affect our brains. The participants in this study were all healthy and not obese, and hooked up to gastric tubes which would be supplying their body with mystery-food solutions throughout the test. The (pretty brave) participants didn't know if they were going to be receiving sugar, salt, fat, protein or tequila. As they were receiving the solutions, they were frequently asked to rate their emotional responses on a scale of one (crap) to nine (happy!) with five being neutral, and simultaneously were all having their brains scanned with MRI. Intense.[42]

The participants were also played pieces of music deemed to be either neutral or sad, and shown images also deemed to be either neutral or sad. The results showed that the introduction of fat *before* being exposed to 'sad' images or music helped to decrease the 'sad' responses in the participants. Wey! But the introduction of fat *during* the 'sad' ambush left participants feeling unsatiated and without a feeling of fullness. The MRIs showed that the sensitive response areas in the brain were the hippocampus (our judging panel) and the hypothalamus (Kylie Minogue).

Hmm, can't really ignore the fact that the study showed that eating fat **when** you're sad does nothing to help you, though. Curse you, science, who invited you anyway?

There's an argument that we're faced with a chicken and egg situation here, but more like a fried chicken and a sad Easter-egg face. What comes first, people wonder: poor diet or depression?

Gut feelings and happy hormones

The majority of our serotonin is, in fact, produced in our gastro-intestinal tract. *Record scratch* I know, right? Up to 90 per cent of our serotonin is made in our digestive tract. It's the same as the serotonin that we make in our brain but made from different types of cells and with different functions compared to brain-made serotonin. Serotonin in our digestive tract regulates function and movements of the bowel – which explains why the Depression Poops are 'a thing', and also – and I found this part fascinating – serotonin in our digestive tract helps us to feel full while we're eating.

Thus, I think it's fair to say that a lack of serotonin inside ya could mean a lack of control around your eating habits, and difficulty knowing whether or not you're feeling full; this is of course a very common issue in those who've suffered from bulimia or other eating disorders.

There are studies that claim serotonin is 'nature's appetite suppressant' and that it's triggered in your body when you eat carbs.[43]

The relationship between our guts and our brains has been pretty well documented, and it's known that they're always chatting to each other via our vagus nerve (which runs from your brain through your face and thorax to the abdomen).

The microbes our bodies need to produce serotonin naturally come from the amino acid called tryptophan. This particular amino acid is found in a whole bunch of non-vegan foods such as fish, poultry, milk, eggs and cheese (particularly cottage cheese), but also in peanuts, pumpkin seeds, tofu, soy and sesame seeds.

Alas, scientists haven't found any direct links between eating foods rich with tryptophan resulting in improved mental health (there are some soft links to increased sleepiness as a result of digesting tryptophan, but more research is still needed)[44] – so put down that bucket of sesame seeds. Also, increased gut serotonin doesn't necessarily lead to increased mental wellbeing. If your gut is poisoned with a bacteria like, say, E. coli, it will naturally produce a (quite literal) crap-load of serotonin to help you, er, empty out your guts and remove the poison. I've never found food poisoning to lull me into a particularly euphoric state, but each to their own.

A different brand of food influencers have done their bit to launch a scientifically unstable representation of the 'clean eating' movement on social media. Many claim that their move to a diet of fresh berries and rabbit food has completely rid them of mental strain and physical aches, and now they do rooftop yoga at dawn every day before eating a small teaspoon of moondust. This is the 'clean eating' diet taken to a damaging extreme, and has been shown to be behind a saddening increase of orthorexia – a condition where the sufferer will go out of their way to avoid eating foods they conceive to be unhealthy, while maintaining an (unhealthy) extreme focus on only consuming healthy foods. The sufferer will obsessively avoid certain foods due to their alleged association with negative effects on their health, and often without any actual medical advice whatsoever.

Being aware of the nutritional value of your food isn't a bad thing, obvs, but people with orthorexia will become consumed with nutritional information to the extent that they end up doing their bodies way more harm than good.

It's easy to see how this can be provoked and encouraged in the world of shiny smoothie bowls and hemp-flaxseed-pixie-dust-milkshakes we see on social media. I'm glad I don't live in LA. Orthorexia is still being studied, and seems to fall somewhere around the point of a hellish mixture of an eating disorder and obsessive compulsive disorder.

Beat, the UK's eating disorder charity, says that orthorexia 'is not currently recognized in a clinical setting as a separate eating disorder, so someone who visited the doctor with the symptoms would not be officially diagnosed with "orthorexia", although the term may be brought up when discussing their illness'.[45]

Deakin University in Australia actually has a Food & Mood Centre (I knew it was a good name), and the director of the department has completed some astonishing research. Felice Jacka, also President of the International Society for Nutritional Psychiatry Research, has dedicated her career to focusing on the connection between nutrition and mental health, which is ever so helpful for this chapter. Thanks, Felice.

Felice Jacka studied a group of 250 people in 2015, and through her testing she found that adults with unhealthier diets actually presented with *smaller left hippocampal volume* than the adults who ate better.[46]

SMALLER HIPPOCAMPI as a direct result of eating crap. Uh oh.

For a trial published in 2017, she studied sixty-seven participants who were all experiencing depression at the time.[47] She randomly split the group into two and gave each one different types of support, to measure the effect it had on their mental health. The first group was called 'the befriending group' and acted as the control, the second group was the 'diet group'.

The befriending group regularly met with members of the research team to discuss subjects enjoyable to them (that didn't include anything emotional or related to mental health). The 'diet group' received the same social support with these conversations, but also a 'dietary intervention' (woah) that involved them following a typically Mediterranean diet plan for the three months that the study took place.

At the end of the study all the participants had their levels of mental and physical health assessed. Another three months later (so six months after the study began) the researchers followed up with a phone call to each participant for one more health assessment.

TA-DA: The 'diet group' won. 'At the end of the trial, a third of those in the dietary support group met criteria for remission of major depression, compared to 8 per cent of those in the social support group.

'These results were not explained by changes in physical activity or body weight, but were closely related to the extent of dietary change. In other words, those who improved their diet the most experienced the greatest benefit to their depression.'

Of course, this study was relatively small with just sixty-seven participants, but it backs up my plan to move to the coast and live the dream life in the Med, so I've included it here. Maybe you can join me and we can live on a sad little island together and eat yogurt.

Vitamin SEA

Right, so we're eating like a Mediterranean chef – but only for eight hours a day – and we're not following unqualified nutritionists and food bloggers on Instagram who are telling us to put unicorn dust on our cereal. But what about all the noise around vitamin deficiency and its link to our gloom?

The internet's full of conflicting advice about vitamin B12, vitamin D and selenium – all commonly found in meat, which other studies and practitioners have told us to avoid... so... huh?

Some studies say that B12 significantly decreases symptoms of depression when accompanied with antidepressants,[48] some say it does bugger all.[49]

Essentially – and frustratingly – this, like most things, comes down to each individual. There doesn't seem to be a one-size-fits-all approach to improving your mental health through your diet. The closest anyone has come to solving that conundrum has shown that we should eat like they do in the Med, which isn't impossible, but good-quality food is often out of reach for a lot of us as it can be pretty pricey. Luckily this is where our nemesis and lover, the internet, can help again, as it's full of 'budget-friendly ways to follow a Mediterranean diet' and I'll certainly be trying to give it a go.

Some things worth trying to improve your mood with food:

- Remember that half the nutrition from food is going up to the party in your brain. Growing a healthier brain will be a lot quicker if you feed it more vegetables and fruits and less beer and pork scratchings. We want the Serena Williams of brains, not the Homer Simpson.
- BUT. Don't be mean to yourself and refuse to have a biscuit because it's unhealthy. If it will help you feel better momentarily, eat it.
- Convenience is your friend. We know that depression saps the energy out of you, and you're hardly going to feel like making a fresh Mediterranean delight for every meal. Batch-cook when you can, and look into healthy 'instant' options like pre-packed salads, veg, soups and deliveries. It's all very well going to a market to virtuously purchase fresh fruit and award-winning veg, but not so great if all your giant marrows go mouldy in the fridge.

- As usual, take advantage of the time when you feel less awful. If you find yourself having a good moment or hour or few days, note down what you've been eating and drinking so you can have an informed look. I know, it sounds basic, but it could be a good list to look at when you're feeling deathly again in an attempt to get some good health back into you. In the same breath it's worth noting down what you've consumed ahead of you falling into the gloom trap, but I realize it's hard to do anything at all when the gloom is all-consuming.
- Eat some ice cream. I have highlighted its benefits and really will judge you if you don't go for it.

The clapbacks

It's infuriating when anyone tries to give you dietary advice, and immediately makes you think of the last 'bad' thing you ate. Short of having a basket of squishy tomatoes to throw at this person, maybe they'd be better responded to with:

'There is no medical proof that fasting in any way helps mental health, or physical health for that matter. Shall we go get some chips?'

'I'm actually saving up to move to the south of Spain in order to eat a medically recommended diet. Got any cash?'

CHAPTER 12

Ever think you should cut back on the drink, darl?

OK, here's the Big One. The one I don't want to write because it means having a proper look at drinking habits, and I can hardly bang on about how 'alcohol is a depressant – so oi! Put down that pinot grigio!' – when I turn to alcohol as self-medication all the damn time.

Insanity is when you do something over and over again and keep expecting it to have different results than the last time you did it. Does it count as insanity if you keep filling up your glass as you're enjoying the booze buzz and how it's clouding up your brain, you're enjoying how it's magically making you appear social, chatty and like nothing is wrong, and you're enjoying the feeling of your horrible, dark thoughts blurring into a mess that you can't read anymore?

Drinking is a gamble if you're depressed. Sometimes the sauce will do exactly what I want it to do and sometimes when you drink to try to stop yourself thinking and try to numb your pain, all it does is aggravate it. So you drink more, because it's not working, and more still, because the pain isn't dulling, and it eventually tips you down a hole so deep you think you'll never claw yourself back out.

Then there's the aftermath. The Booze Blues. The Beer Fear. The Dooms. Hangxiety, and other catchy names we've given it to try and casually gloss over the fact that we've willingly poured vast quantities of a substance into ourselves that is known to make us depressed. Even people who don't suffer from clinical depression will feel depressed after a big night on the razzle dazzle, and to top it all off, we've paid VAST EXPENSE for the experience! We! Are! So! Thick!

But yes, I will have a gin martini, thanks. Dry, bit of lemon, lovely stuff. If alcohol was invented today there is no fucking way it would be legal. But then, if alcohol wasn't around today, how different the world would be...Women's bathrooms in nightclubs would be empty of embracing, toiletry sharing and tough love about a wrong'un who happens to be in the same bar. Cities on a Friday night would be abuzz with the low thrum of locals enjoying a lovely cup of mint tea. James Bond would drink tomato juice. Wetherspoon's wouldn't exist. Ireland would be empty and St Patrick forgotten. Jesus would have left the water as water and there'd be far less interest in France.

Also, maybe there would be fewer suicides.

This part is difficult to address because I love alcohol. I am regularly *praised for the amount of alcohol I can drink* (British culture truly celebrates the wrong things). People who can 'really put the booze away' are generally, I have found, fucked up. You don't need a medical degree to know that while you're suffering with depression and taking antidepressants as *well* as trying a whole host of other stuff to try to squash the depression demons, drinking alcohol, *an actual depressant,* is like giving the depression demons CPR and a fresh pack of batteries, cancelling out all the other work you're trying to do.

I admirably read the stories of people who have made the bold (and undoubtedly wise) step to become sober to support their health. I think, 'That's great for you and I applaud you, good woman, but ha! Obviously, that's not what I need to do because I don't need alcohol to enjoy myself.'

Yeah, well, you don't need a car to take you from A to B but it certainly gets you there quicker than walking, doesn't it?

I love drinking. I love drinking endless bottles of red wine while out for dinner somewhere with soft lighting and squashy seats. I love drinking frozen margaritas in the sunshine, in a race to finish them before the ice has melted and 'ruined it'. I love drinking gin and tonics with massive slices of grapefruit at summer barbecues, or having a fruit cider as the first drink at a festival when you're hungover 'to take the edge off'. I love the arrival of a cold, spicy Bloody Mary and some hot salty chips, and the first taste of a cold, frothy beer on holiday. I love gins in tins on trains, and little plastic glasses on planes. I love how you always toast your 'first Baileys of the season' because it's 'really Christmas now', and how you always drink limoncello in an Italian restaurant even though it tastes like medicine.

I love the moment on a night out when everyone thinks shots of tequila are an excellent idea, and how there's always one person who has to have a sambuca instead because tequila makes them gag. I love tinnies in the park. I love the split-second of eye contact with a co-worker at lunch when the server asks what you'd like to drink and you both pretend that you've suddenly succumbed to the surprise thought of having a wine.

But alcohol doesn't love us in return. Alcohol is the ultimate fuckboi. Alcohol makes us think that it's showing us a good time and then leaves us in the shit to fester. A woman called Vanessa told me:

Alcohol is a massive trigger for a decline in my mental health. Even just one or two drinks will make me feel a lot worse the next day. People have often talked about 'hangxiety', but when you have poor mental health this is so much worse. I will feel extremely emotional; my anxiety will intensify and often I will have a panic attack. I feel extremely alone, which then sends my thoughts on a downward spiral.

Alcohol makes us fall over, injure ourselves and lose possessions. Alcohol makes people immune to the word no, and emboldens already despicable, lecherous types to really try to push it with someone who wants nothing to do with them, or even push, punch or otherwise abuse them. Alcohol makes us violent. Alcohol makes us forget entire sections of evenings that we want to remember. Alcohol makes us late for work, makes us stink of a pub drip-tray and makes even our classiest friends vomit on themselves.

Alcohol impairs our judgement. Alcohol is why there are 'beer goggles' and people who are 'six gins in' (only hot when you've had six gins, just to be clear). Alcohol can make the truth come out and also pushes out floods of lies. Alcohol makes some people wet the bed. Alcohol takes away entire days that you had great plans for, that are instead reduced to remaining horizontal and in pain and full of fear and regret and vomit. Alcohol can poison you. Alcohol can kill you if you drink too much at once. Alcohol is often a poison of choice when people do choose to kill themselves on purpose.

Oh, alcohol.

When you're drunk, you can't feel your pain as much. When you're drunk, you feel happy! Fun! Even actually JOYFUL sometimes. It's a window into a wild other life without depression, and you just need to keep on drinking to keep up the buzz. But then it gets to the point when you can't stop, and you're chasing the buzz for hours when everyone else is off home to bed and to be spooned by their partner, and you're at a bar on your own in Soho at 5 a.m. and you've bought a prostitute drinks and chips so you'll have some company. Anything that'll help delay the return to sobriety and 'regular life' for as long as possible.

When you're drunk, so drunk, sometimes you black out. You can't feel anything in the present and you can't remember anything in the past. I read about it being called a 'mini suicide', and, well… quite.

I spoke to a gal called Maisy, who told me that she thinks her drinking is actually a form of self-harm. This comparison from her hit me like a slap in the face, and I totally agree with her. It's damaging, it's painful, it's going to be awful the next day, and we can't stop doing it because it gives us a guilty release at the time. Maisy also told me:

I have always been more inclined to self-harm in long-term painful ways, which I guess leads me on to my relationship with alcohol. I've used alcohol and drugs for a long time in order to have some short-term solace from my mental health issues. Being blackout drunk gives me an evening off from my constant anxiety and depression, and I've often used drugs as a way to place myself into social situations and feel comfortable talking to people. The worst thing with the alcohol is my hangovers afterwards (that often last at least two days), and the anxiety that ensues as I'm suffering with the hangover. I'm still struggling with alcohol today.

I hear that.

I often wonder what I would do if I didn't drink alcohol. Sure, I'd keep a cleaner apartment and read more books and probably eat a lot more healthily (OK, that does sound pretty good...), but, like, where would I *go*? I can barely think of a social activity that appeals to me that doesn't revolve around drinking.

There's a security blanket that comes with drinking alcohol, and people feel nervous and exposed if you take it away. If you head to the pub to meet friends and order a lime and soda because 'I'm gonna stay off it tonight' people will look at you like you've come to their house for Sunday lunch and slapped their gran in the face.

'But WHY?' they'll ask. 'Ah come one, one little glass won't hurt!' Dré once committed to three months without drinking, and despite the fact that he still went out with his friends to pretty much every social gathering, and stayed out until the last Ubers were taking everyone home, people still told him, 'Let us know when you're not being boring, yeah, and we'll go for a real night out.'

People get nervous if they find out that they're drinking and you're not. It's like you've given them a vial of truth serum and they're terrified about what's going to come out while you sit there, judging them and taking notes, tutting to yourself as they stumble over their words and tell you a story they already told you a few hours ago. I think it was A. A. Gill who wrote about the fact that if you're not drinking, there is never a conversation-ally rich reason to stay out after everyone's finished their fourth drink – and he was right.

Also – and I'm not making excuses here (or maybe I am) – can we have a moment for the absolute scandal of the non-alcoholic gin that costs the same amount of money as the gin that makes you cry to strangers? What, pray tell, is the point of that? If I'm paying £10 for a drink, I want to at least feel something. But that's the problem, isn't it? Feelings.

Psychotherapists know a lot about feelings, so I spoke to John-Paul Davies about our urge to purge on the fizzy pops when we're feeling dark. Don't worry, he told me:

> It's absolutely understandable that we drink to feel better in the short term when we're depressed.
>
> Drinking changes our stressed or numb state by releasing rewarding chemicals like dopamine, that feel good in the short term. As humans, we're programmed to choose the shortest way possible to do anything, and therefore come with an inbuilt, natural preference for alcohol's quick relief.
>
> Of course, the trouble with temporarily rewarding substances like alcohol is that they'll never provide anything other than short-term relief and they change nothing else in our life that could help alleviate the depression. Unless we learn other ways of feeling calm and alive, as we also know, abuse of alcohol can set up an addiction that makes depression worse, triggering more drinking to temporarily feel better and catching us in a vicious circle.

OK, please don't feel guilty about your affections for booze after reading that. I'm choosing instead to focus on his words about learning other ways of '**feeling calm and alive**'. I've never thought about it like that before. I feel so hardwired to go for a glass of wine if I'm stressed, I've probably convinced myself it's the only thing that works. There are, obvs, other things that can make us feel calm and alive SURELY. For me I know that travel is one of them, and being outside somewhere green. Alas, these aren't as easy to do on a Friday night (who am I kidding, a Monday lunchtime) as it is to just go to a bar.

My Internet Friend (we talk on Twitter) Dave, has an interesting way of looking at it. He told me:

> *I firmly believe that I have nothing left to achieve when it comes to drinking, I have some of the greatest drinking stories anyone could have; I have gone out drinking in Dublin and ended up in Wales, I've gone straight from a nightclub to an airport to fly to Spain to keep the party going, and blagged my way backstage at everything from gigs to golf championships, so I pretty much don't need to drink to make any crazy new memories.*

A good point, enhanced further by the fact that when we drink to the state of excess and 'mini suicide', which we tend to do, we often can't remember anything anyway. There's no point drinking 'to see what fun will happen' – because we know what will happen. Oblivion.

I'm seriously considering going sober, but the thought honestly terrifies me because I am not fun without booze. I am Fun Bobby from *Friends* with less impressive hair. Plus, as mentioned, I fucking love alcohol.

Even if there was magical medication that would make

depression a distant memory but with the one, ONE condition that it would only work if you didn't have any alcohol – would I take it? Would you?

It's interesting (read: a behaviour indicative of alcoholic dependency and fear of what life would be like without a boozy crutch to rely on) to watch everyone try to tread the careful, ginger dance around booze and medication, in order to find the very precise and exact balance that allows them to continue on the slosh while not ruining the intended effects of the meds. We all love alcohol so much – until we don't – that we'll 'experiment' over and over again even though we know it's doomed to failure.

We try to make the art of mixing drinks and (prescription) drugs into an exact science. 'If I start drinking and then take my meds half an hour later with some water and paracetamol then I should be OK for another two hours when I'll take another pill and then as long as I do five star jumps before bed I'll be fine.'

This is clearly entirely pointless if you're on antidepressants, isn't it, because there's no science and YOU'RE JUST RUINING IT.

Or, *au contraire*, are your antidepressants making it all more fun? An unexpected side effect of my antidepressants is that they have almost totally and entirely eliminated hangovers altogether, which is wildly dangerous, considering my reliance on alcohol and willingness to test just how much I can drink before the meds crack and a hangover bleeds into my head. 'Even if I start feeling better I'm gonna keep taking them just for the no hangovers!' I have been known to squawk, but I'm hardly gonna get better if I keep supping on martini glasses of gloom, am I?

I probably would take that magical medication after all.

But alcoholics are always having a Carlsberg at 8 a.m. and wearing fingerless gloves, like Fagin, and mumbling things about the war. Alcoholics don't have jobs and apartments with fairy lights. Alcoholics don't light scented candles and get annoyed when it looks like their plant's gone a bit brown.

Bryony Gordon has a wonderfully insightful book about her relationship with alcohol and eventual sobriety (it's called *Glorious Rock Bottom*), and she has said that her park bench was her sofa, but surely it doesn't count if you've done the sophisticated thing and gone to the effort of putting your wine *into a glass*, right?

Look, I like to have a joke (attempt), but I know I'm not an alcoholic, in all seriousness. I don't need it to get through the day, and I don't drink in the mornings... unless it's Christmas, or brunch.

But sure, I have alcoholic tendencies. I think most people in our generation do, right? We get to the point on a night out where there's no 'off' switch. When you've had so much to drink already that suddenly you're dying of thirst, and when you get home a lot more than half-cut you instantly reach for a bottle of wine 'to keep things going' or you end up wandering the streets with the only other two people from your group who are just as sad and desperate and as scared of going to their homes alone as you are, to end up in a strange bar with three customers, £10 pints and the big light on. But booze! Hey! They're still serving! Nice one.

Yeah, there have been times when I've put a bottle of wine *back on the shelf after not finishing it all in one night*, but there have also been times when I've stayed in alone and drunk five (five) bottles of wine to myself in an attempt to get so drunk that I sleep through the entirety of the next day and just keep skipping forward (the wine was super-cheap, otherwise I would have had spirits).

Sure, there have been times when I've made myself a cocktail and thought, 'Nah, not really feeling it,' and called it a night after that, but there have also been nights when I've drunk the house out of vodka and been woken up on the sofa at 7 a.m. by Dré getting ready to go to work, looking at me with concerned pity as I scratch the crusty dribble from my cheek.

Life's all about balance!

Ahem.

It's a very British/Irish thing that we all tolerate drinking so much and make blithe jokes about alcohol consumption that are actually just honest accounts of what we did last night, but everybody laughs because it's so absurd. In most other parts of Europe they serve beer IN MCDONALD'S. Can you imagine the absolute raw hell that would ensue if there was beer in Maccy's in the UK?

When I speak to friends from outside the UK and say that I started swigging capfuls of vodka with my friends at about thirteen, and got kicked out of a twelve-year-old's disco party because I'd stolen a bottle of Stella Artois from the pantry (but, being twelve, hadn't stolen a bottle opener, so was found by a peeved parent as I clumsily tried to open the bottle on the railings outside the community hall…), they are somewhat shocked.

Speak to anyone else who came of age in the UK and they won't bat an eyelid. *Skins* was tame compared to what we got up to when we were pretending to be at a sleepover. By fifteen we all had our 'drinks of choice' (I will never let Dré forget that his drink of choice at the time, as confessed on one of those email quiz things, was a very 2002-esque Malibu and lemonade).

We drank as teens, but it wasn't to excess, I don't think, it just didn't take us as much to get drunk then and we only had £20 from our waitressing jobs so had to buy (or swipe from parents) the strongest, cheapest stuff that would do the trick. I was once grounded for weeks when my mum found a plastic water bottle in my bedside drawer that I'd filled with 'a little bit of this, a little bit of that' from about fifteen of my parents' finest spirits. I still owe my dad a bottle of seventeen-year-aged Glenmorangie after I ruined his bottle-that-was-being-saved by slugging a bit into my over-potent mix to drink down the park.

I remember feeling incredibly depressed as a teenager, but then, aren't all teenagers? I remember sitting in my bedroom and listening to Linkin Park (who really, like, understood me) and thinking about how much their lyrics about wanting to die really spoke to me.

Teen years are a headfuck anyway with all the extra doses of hormones bubbling around you. Add to that a few attempted suicides from friends (one with live commentary on the phone to me as he did it – thank God my middle-class parents had a second phone line at the time, which I could use to call the ambulance to his house. Usually it was reserved strictly for the internet or as a double-phone-attack on the Boyzone concert ticketing offices from the years 1994–1999).

I remember when my friends started experimenting with stuff that wasn't booze or weed, but a bit more serious sounding. They'd got it, of course, from the older boys we were hanging out with who at the time we all thought were incredibly edgy and cool, but with hindsight were sad and creepy to choose to spend their time with a bunch of fourteen-year-olds when they were all nearing twenty-one.

I got a phone call one night from two of my best friends who had taken acid and thought they were dead. Turns out they were stuck in a very white, bright bathroom, which they understood as being 'the other side', and it seemed like about six terrifying hours passed before they realized they were, in fact, alive and just gathered around a bog. 'Ha,' I thought, 'look at them on hard drugs. I am a superior queen who shall not dabble in such things and get myself in such a state.'

Flash forward three years to me drinking so much vodka I passed out in the bathroom of one of those friends (oh, how the tables had turned), didn't know where I was and convinced my parents (who were worried sick on the phone) that I'd been drugged and kidnapped. You don't need 'harder stuff' to mess yourself up. Alcohol is hard enough.

Turns out, though, that if you really don't want to drink when you're on a night out you basically have to prepare yourself to be asked about it three times, and then it's done. The first 'What?! You're not having a proper drink?' will be followed by a 'Come on, mate, have some fun, are you sure?' and when you say, 'I'm sure, drinking makes me really miserable these days,' you're likely to only get a 'decided to have some fun yet?' on the next round, and that'll be it. As much as I hate to admit it, saying no might be one of the best things that you can actually do for your mental health.

The clapbacks

I honestly don't know what to say here, apart from, 'Yeah, probably should cut down.'

Oops.

CHAPTER 13

Just 'man up', mate

Are you eye-rolling? I'm eye-rolling. This is one of the worst.

We've all seen the high-street children's clothing sections that still have T-shirts 'for boys' that say something like 'When I grow up I'll be a scientist' and T-shirts 'for girls' that say 'YAY FLOWERS'. We remember being told that if a boy hits a girl it's because he likes her, and if a boy cries he's being a sissy (but girls crying was fine).

Young boys grow up being told that anything emotional – besides anger – is not 'manly' and should be suppressed. Reading this sentence won't be the first time you've come across comments like 'man up', 'don't be a fairy' and 'you cry/throw/run/breathe like a girl', which will almost always have been directed at men. Seemingly casual 'banter' (vom at that word) like this means that a lot of boys grow up into men who are embarrassed, ashamed or unaware of how to express emotional feelings beyond those that portray them as strong or dominant in any given situation. Any sign of weakness is taken as a sign of being 'less of a man'.

Of course, everyone carries a large Santa sack of complex

emotions regardless of what gender they identify as, but it's men in particular who are conditioned to think that if they or other men actually admit to feeling them or express them in any way, they're lesser. So, as a result, a lot of men bottle up all of the emotion that they're ashamed of and don't address it at all.

By being raised in a world where they're not allowed to have feelings, many men are now exploding internally with the pressure of the emotion they don't feel able to express. This can manifest externally in a whole host of symptoms, including men retreating inwards and taking their own lives – which it does. All the time.

Suicide is the biggest killer of men in the UK.[50]

In the UK, men are three times more likely to die by suicide than women. In Ireland it's four times more.[51]

Our men are killing themselves, and, as a cis woman, I feel like I can't really say much more on the subject apart from to rant about how the patriarchy is damaging for everyone of all genders, and equality for all is not just about having more parity and inclusion of genders and ethnicities in boardrooms, in media and in schools. Equality for all can save lives. So I've enlisted some insightful men to share their experiences of mental health struggles they may have had due to everybody's favourite jazz-handsy buzz phrase, toxic masculinity.

If you've managed to avoid hearing this phrase up until now, it's important to highlight that toxic masculinity does not mean that all men are asbestos, instead it refers to the 'traditional gender roles' applied to men throughout their lives from when they were very small boys. The phrase is calling out how toxic the *traditional notion of masculinity* is, where men have been taught by society that they should limit their emotions and put on a facade of bravado to become a chest-beating alpha male.

This man is 'butch' and 'macho' and surrounds himself with things like… trucks and, er… The Rock. This man would never be friends with a gay guy, let alone be gay himself, are you MAD? He loves TITS TITS TITS and REALLY FAST CARS and CANS OF LAGER and COMPLAINING ABOUT CARS and TITS and the PRICE OF CANS OF LAGER.

Side note: the aforementioned Dwayne 'The Rock' Johnson has spoken publicly about his struggles with depression, telling the media how at one point he was constantly crying and unable to stop. Following the publication of the interview, he tweeted that it's important for 'us dudes' to talk about mental health, as 'we have a tendency to keep it in. You're not alone.'

Toxic masculinity is a persuasion that if a male has any feeling more delicate than the red mist of rage, they can't be 'a real man'. It's not just referring to existing as a man, it's the notion that men are only 'proper manly men' if they're straight, muscular, emotionless and know the names of every team in the Premier League and of various types of screwdriver.

This heartbreakingly seems to be especially embedded into men aged over fifty, a lot of whom feel unable to talk about their mental health struggles because it would reveal the 'lesser man' behind the Wizard of Oz's big shiny green facade. A fifty-seven-year-old pal (who would like to remain anonymous, so let's call him Steve here) told me that this is 'especially the case in the corporate world. Businessmen keep up a hard front, and there's no way anyone would ever feel comfortable saying that they get down sometimes. If an esteemed colleague said that they cry a lot, his peers would wonder what the hell they were doing trusting him with their professional matters.' How utterly tragic.

I spoke to a less anonymous friend, Andrew, who is also in the Boomer generation (parents of millennials, largely) and hasn't felt able to talk about his mental health for the precise reasons of being both a man and a father. He told me:

I am nearing sixty and have suffered from periods of depression for most of my life. My mother and my sister also suffer from it as well. I have never been able to talk about it. Other men don't want to talk about any health issues, while as the breadwinner and father of children I've always wanted to appear strong and reliable. Talking with my middle son (who I have been trying to help with his mood swings), he told me I have always come across as so controlled that he never noticed I was stressed or depressed – although he does notice that at times I do drink more. I don't think as a man of my generation or responsibilities anybody has been interested in my mental health, or that I have a venue for discussing it.

Younger generations seem to be far more open to talking about mental health, but that doesn't mean it's without its challenges and prejudices. The phrase 'man up' is still very much in use, alongside 'grow some balls' and 'don't be such a pussy'. Steve told me:

The concept of 'traditional masculinity' is a big part of men not talking or opening up about their mental health issues. I've found it incredibly hard to open up and talk about things, even to my wife and to close family members. We were brought up in that masculine storyline: it's just not what blokes do. Manly men are meant to 'man up and carry on' without 'showing signs of weakness'. I started to suffer from depression and anxiety about four years ago. Initially I did shrug it off, but then more recently realized I really did need help.

I finally went to my GP, who referred me to some local services that could help me. I'm also doing an online CBT course where I still get my own, dedicated practitioner, and it's really helping me.

Seeking medical help is a huge step for anyone suffering from mental health struggles, and talking about said struggles with people you actually see in your 'real life' is even harder. But – especially with men – these conversations can provide crucial support for other fellas who are struggling and have never felt able to open up about it, look for help or even 'admit it' to themselves.

Another guy I spoke with, Caspar, seriously suffered with clinical depression a few years ago. He told me:

It's a well-known fact that suicide in men is far higher than in women, because we men tend to hide it far more, and feel like it's a sign of weakness or shame, or that we can't cope with life's challenges.

As men, we don't really talk to our mates about how we feel emotionally, as we feel we'll probably be told that we'll 'just have to get on with it' or 'have a beer, mate, and you'll be fine'.

But I discovered that whenever I opened up about my depression, it also helped other guys to say, 'Actually, me too, mate, and I have suffered for years.' More men speaking up will be crucial for other men to feel they, too, can say that they do not feel OK.'

It's still so difficult for many men to feel like they can open up about their mental health, and I've included a list of great resources in the appendix if you or someone you know could do with some support. Maybe show them the list if you don't feel like they'd be open to talking to you about mental health in more depth just yet.

Talking about your state of mind, both for men and women, is still largely seen as a weakness, and it's up to all of us to start discussions about mental health and show that talking about depression, anxiety or anything else that might be going on is not going to put the lid on any career or romantic progression in your life. It might even save your life.

Dré, lovely man that he is, shared a sad but hopeful story of his own:

There were many times as a kid when I was told to 'man up', but I don't think I was ever actually told what a 'man' should be. I wasn't really sure what I was doing that was beneath the definition of a man and what I should do to raise myself to that standard. I wasn't even told why it was so important that I be one, other than that was what was expected of me, so I had to do it. Whatever it was.

If I was afraid, I was told to 'grow some balls', which meant to me that if I feel fear then I'm not really a man. So, as a kid I was left to connect the dots that by feeling less you're somehow more of a 'man'. I can remember in school someone biting through their tongue because they got hit in the face with a baseball, but what I also remember is that what people cared about more was the fact that he cried while he was led away by the teacher. You couldn't even cry if you'd almost bitten your tongue off. I was laughed at in primary school for crying when I needed to get five stitches in my mouth after being accidentally kicked in the face.

Thankfully my experience with this is different today. The big difference I've found is that my male friends and I have started talking to each other. Like actually talking talking, about our actual feelings.

Honestly, I cannot emphasize enough how strange this felt at first. In my experience, spending time with my male friends has always consisted of talking about anything other than how you felt. It took me a long time to realize that we wouldn't even ask each other how we were when we'd meet up. 'How's it going?' would be replied to with a 'Yeah, how's it going?' and the conversation moved on quickly. Whether or not this was a societal pressure or just more personally how I interacted with my friends, I'm not sure.

What surprised me when I first started to talk about how I felt was just how much my mates really wanted to listen, and to share their feelings themselves. It felt a bit like, 'Oh, we're actually allowed to talk about this stuff? Why didn't anyone tell me?'

I still have mates who will never talk about how they're feeling, or will use jokes to deflect it, but since I've started to open up and talk about my feelings, they've started to do the same and sometimes it looks like a weight has been visibly lifted from their shoulders.

I think it might've even saved a mate's life.

OK, so this started off sadly and did make me cry thinking of poor cute little child-Dré being laughed at for his tears, but it ends so encouragingly. I love to think of guys 'breaking the barrier' (cheesy sounding, but true) by talking about feelings with their friends, and seeing others follow suit.

The Mental Health Foundation reports that around one in eight men in the UK have a mental health problem and that men are less likely to talk about their mental health than women.[52] Some famous men have been talking about their experiences with depression, though, which is helpful.

- **Jon Hamm** (of *Mad Men* fame) said that he was in bad shape when struggling with chronic depression, and that having therapy helped him enormously. 'It gives you another perspective when you are so lost in your own spiral, your own bullshit,' he said.
- **Rob Delaney** from *Catastrophe* has been open about his recovery from alcoholism and depression, saying, 'I suffer

from all the classical negative, stereotypical thoughts, where I think, "I don't need any help." The fact is, it is strong to ask for help. It is strong to say, 'OK, there's a problem that I don't have the resources to fix myself." [...] Get help. And that means walking into an emergency room if necessary. Ideally, you'll catch it before you get to that point, but don't be embarrassed if it comes to that.'

- **Hugh Laurie** said that his depression 'affected everything – my family and friends. I was a pain in the arse to have around. I was miserable and self-absorbed.'

- **Bruce Springsteen** has worked with his mental health to get it into a place where he manages it with medication. 'I have come close enough to [mental illness] where I know I am not completely well myself. I've had to deal with a lot of it over the years, and I'm on a variety of medications that keep me on an even keel; otherwise I can swing rather dramatically and... just... the wheels can come off a little bit.'

My friend Nick told me what he really thinks:

The pressure on men around showing signs of what may have once been considered weakness is definitely decreasing. However, I'm very aware that my socioeconomic background and the social circles I operate in mean that I'm in a privileged situation both in terms of education about things like this and acceptance from my peers.

In fact, I feel very lucky that my experiences of opening up to men have all been very positive. If anything, the men in my life I was most worried about being honest with actually turned out to be the most accepting of and receptive to the conversation. As a teenager, I definitely experienced the pressure of having to 'man up' – from adults – but nothing like this has ever been said to me explicitly as an adult myself. It can be hard to tell whether it's my personality that led me to taking a while to open up about my depression or whether I have internalized the societal norms around masculinity from a young age which led me to develop those tendencies in the first place.

I really think that today, male mental health is being treated a lot more seriously – not yet as honestly, openly and as seriously as it should be, perhaps, but it certainly seems like it's a more open place for people to approach the subject.

So how do we drive change? I truly think that the most effective ways of changing how people think and behave, and introducing compassionate education, is to have conversations with those closest to you. Challenge your friends who make racist, sexist or homophobic comments, who tell other men to 'man up' or make jokes about men having feelings being lesser than men who hide theirs away. Don't just awkwardly laugh over it and say 'not cool' – do more. Ignoring them won't change anything.

A few men told me what's recently encouraged them to speak out about their mental health, whether to friends or therapists. Unsurprisingly, it was still difficult to get responses from men on the subject of mental health, and a few came back to me with 'I don't need to talk, I just have a spliff, WAHEY' jokes. There's more work to be done.

- 'A friend asked another friend about their mental health in a friendly, open setting. It made us all more encouraged to talk about it.'
- 'Male public figures talking about it in a relatable way makes it seem more normal.'
- 'All the media noise about men being able to talk about their feelings... it actually helped.'
- 'Having friends who talked about theirs made me feel like I could talk about mine, so much so that I then went to a therapist. Having a safe space to discuss it even if I don't need to, just knowing it's there, is a huge help.'

Trisha, a teacher who has taught in London, Beijing and now Singapore, tells me that things are looking up for the next generation of guys, too:

In Beijing and Singapore, too, we have school counsellors come into the students' lessons to deliver the wellbeing curriculum, and talk specifically about anxiety and depression and dealing with stress. A lot of our students visit the counsellors for one-on-one sessions when they need, and can contact them by email.

In all three schools I've taught in, mental health has been explicitly taught to pupils through wellbeing lessons in assemblies, and in smaller groups with their form tutor.

But as part of the pastoral care there are many topics leaders need to try and squeeze in such as sex education and revision technique, and sadly available time for anything else can be a bit of a pinch.

I would say with regards to gender it is shifting away from the 'macho man' attitude, certainly from staff. A lot of boys do come and open up, but equally I think pressure still remains from their peers. A lot of the typically 'cool' boys are less likely to open up about their own mental health issues, but equally I see them to be rather respectful of others.

I have to think that this is somewhat helped by the news including statistics and reports around male suicide, and everyone generally taking mental health more seriously these days. If children are being raised without being told to 'man up' or 'grow some balls', then that bodes hugely well for the grown-ups they'll turn into.

Also, as the saying goes: 'If you want to be real tough, grow a vagina. Those things can take a pounding.'

The clapbacks

If someone tells you to 'man up' or 'grow some balls' then there's a chance they're hiding their own insecurities behind ridiculous comments like these, and are saying this stuff to put on a front – your responses might help them see that, actually, there's no place for comments like that anymore. There's also a chance they're just being a douche. Here are some options:

'"Man up" doesn't mean anything. Are you telling me to stop having feelings?'

'How does one go about growing balls, exactly? Can you share any tips? You sound like you must have a very sizeable scrotum.'

'Being a man doesn't mean we can't get sad. I'm trying to open up, please take me seriously.'

'Yeah, I've tried to "get over it" and I've given it time, and it's still a problem. I could really use the support of a friend right now.'

CHAPTER 14

There's a book for that, love

There is. It's this book. End of chapter, thanks for reading. LOLs.

Books will not lift you out of your darkness completely, but (if you can concentrate enough to read, which I presume you can because HELLO, YOU LOVELY READER PERSON), they will provide something on which to focus and not be *as* distracted by the gloom seeping in.

The whole reason I wanted to write something about depression in the first place was because I'd read such great books by other people that made me feel reassured that I wasn't, in fact, going completely mad, and that I definitely wasn't the first person to feel like this. There's never been an entire book that I've consumed and thought 'yep, that's me' on every page (er, apart from this one), but most have offered a handful of 'OMG ME TOO THANK GAWWWD FOR THAT I THOUGHT IT ONLY HAPPENED TO ME' assurances from their insightful pages.

As depression and anxiety throw up an imbalanced cocktail of brain chemistry that we're forced to drink, relaxation and calmness can theoretically help to get that back on track. Whenever I read a passage in a book that I inherently relate to, I'll tear up (because #sadsack) but also feel an immediate jolt of reassurance and calmness.

The notion of a self-help book is a lot more understandable than a self-help film – for now – and like I said, reading books about other people's depression stories and mental health struggles has helped me feel a lot more 'seen'. I'm not saying that a book will cure your depression because LOL, but it can certainly make your longing to be run over by a truck seem more relatable.

When TV presenter Caroline Flack died by suicide, thousands of people donated or bought copies of Matt Haig's depression memoir *Reasons to Stay Alive* and gave them to independent book stores, who had offered to send out copies to anyone who felt they needed one in the wake of such gut-punching news.

Of course, the internet was divided. Some people saw it as a truly kind gesture, of passing on a book to someone who you feel could really benefit from reading it, despite not knowing them at all or even being aware of their existence. Others saw it as an author's way of capitalizing on someone else's death… which is a pretty preposterous accusation, don't you think? The author didn't say, GO, BUY MY BOOK, YOU SAD TWATS, but others recommended it after having read it themselves. It shows the power of a good book, of reading something that makes you say 'oh God, I'm not the only one' and feel so moved that you must press it into the chests of your friends before they go on one more day without reading it.

I have read a lot of books that talk about depression, and have re-read certain passages of them at times I felt like I needed to be reminded that other people have this parade of mind-fuckery, too. I didn't relate to everything Matt said, of course, but the bits that I could recognize in myself gave me such an overwhelming feeling of being inked with a validation stamp that I went on to read more and more depression memoirs, hoping to find that same hit.

Other texts that have made me say 'oh thank fuck for that' include:

Bryony Gordon's *Mad Girl* and *Glorious Rock Bottom*
Sally Brampton's *Shoot the Damn Dog*
Bella Mackie's *Jog On* (this one is really about anxiety much more than depression, though)
Pretty much anything that journalist **Hannah Jane Parkinson** writes about mental health (she is @ladyhaja on Twitter)
Hanya Yanagihara's *A Little Life*
Lori Gottlieb's *Maybe You Should Talk to Someone*
Ruby Wax's *Sane New World*
Marian Keyes's *Rachel's Holiday*

As mentioned earlier in this very book, I wholeheartedly agree with the concept of mind-full-ness: stuffing yourself with books and articles and podcasts and boxsets and culture, and essentially never allowing yourself space to think about how shite you feel.

Fiction in particular can often feel like an injection of some company into an otherwise very solitary existence – though I'm sure you're all too aware that you have to be in a fairly decent place to consume books in the first place, as otherwise you just end up re-reading the same two sentences over and over again in between staring into the middle distance with watery eyes and a heavy head, letting the book drift out of your hand as you retreat under the covers and into the darkness. Thankfully technology has now bequeathed us some podcasts and audiobooks that significantly remove the effort from our side.

Some might argue that filling your mind with distractions is behaviour that echoes that of someone filling their blood with drugs or alcohol; a distraction that offers something else to think about – although I think they're having a laugh (remember laughing?) comparing binge watching a seven-series TV show to being anything like binge drinking seven bottles of Smirnoff.

Researchers at the University of Sussex found that six minutes of reading can reduce your stress levels by up to 68 per cent. The reading effect was higher than going for a walk (a reduction of 42 per cent) or listening to music (61 per cent).[53]

Reading is an activity so different from other media consumption. You have to devote your entire brain space to what's on the page in front of you, or you'll miss something. You can't be absent mindedly scrolling through your phone as you pay half-attention to a book, like you can with a film. You can't be occupied with your dark thoughts when you're keenly following a storyline; it has to be one or the other.

But it's completely true that when you're in the darkest places, reading is impossible. As we're both here on this page, I assume you're in a place where reading can happen for you – or you're reading to find out about how you can support your pal who's depressed. Oh you lovely thing, you.

Depression, in a lot of ways, makes you thick. It buggers your memory and it saps your focus and concentration. Even reading about the riboflavin in your cereal or the sulfates in your shampoo is a momentous task when you're depressed – and both of those suggest you're already exhausted from either forcing yourself to eat or shower anyways. God, it's an illness that turns you into a self-involved, self-loathing, lazy, dense teenager. You are now Harry Enfield's Kevin. This is your life. It's so unfair.

My manager recently got annoyed about me asking a question which she had already told me the answer to 'at least twice now, Kate'. Oops. Because I'm having trouble getting out of bed in the mornings and staying focused every day, my brain is a mess. I'm needing to write down very in-depth notes at work, which are great if I can remember to look at them, so I'm getting written off as a numpty due to the interference with my concentration, focus and short-term memory. I know it's horrible, but in a way I'm glad I'm not the only one. Here are similar experiences from others:

- 'I went through a period of not being able to remember words; I could hardly string a sentence together without forgetting a word. I thought I had early-onset dementia but of course it's a bloody sign of depression!'
- 'Depression did take away my ability to focus. But I also felt so down that I didn't want to focus on anything anyway; everything felt boring and uninteresting, so my mind wandered off someplace else. Actually trying to focus would just remind me I couldn't focus, because I'm depressed, and then I'm in another spiral. I remember it being especially difficult when I was in class, 'cause I couldn't just leave the room for a break so I just sat there trying to disappear.'
- 'It can go either way, so I either obsess about something or I feel paralyzed and unable to do anything. In a particularly bad episode, I can get easily triggered by words, so have to consume media whether that's TV, books or social media in a very conscious way.'
- 'It's most difficult at work when I can struggle to focus for more than ten minutes. Medication helped with that, though.'

- 'When I am at work sometimes, I just can't focus on anything. I read the same sentence over and over again and it doesn't make sense. I put it down to being tired, but I think it's because of the way I am feeling. Waking up in the morning is the hardest but I'm not reading or focusing yet then.'
- 'At one point when my depression got really bad, I couldn't read or write a single sentence. Every time I read a few words, the entire sentence would just evaporate from my mind. It was almost as if I was staring through the screen. Working in a job where I'm constantly responding to emails and drafting huge pieces of copy, you can imagine how frustrating that was for me.'

During the times when you can read, it's easy for books to make you feel a lot more of absolutely nothing. The words chosen so carefully to have an impact have the exact opposite. In English we'd say 'meh', in French they say 'bof'. I think they're both pretty accurate when you remain entirely unmoved and unaffected by anything.

Psychotherapist John-Paul Davies pretty much confirms this with his thoughts on why we find that our reading age drops thirty years when we're depressed. 'When we're depressed, the odds are pretty well stacked against us being able to enjoy reading a book,' he told me. Yes, John-Paul. Yes. He told me:

Being depressed doesn't usually mean we're overwhelmed by feelings, but underwhelmed by them. It's a state where our nervous system is most often under-aroused, where we don't experience the range of emotions we might expect in response to the ups and downs of life. We often read books for pleasure, because of how they make us feel. If we struggle to feel anything when we're reading, we're much less likely to do it, as we're missing the intrinsic reward it used to offer us.

When we're depressed, we also spend little time using our imagination. Depressed thoughts come from the 'threat' part of us, and we're programmed to prioritize them above most other thought types. Threat's role is to identify and respond quickly to aspects of our external environment that it perceives as endangering our physical and/or psychological safety. In terms of real threats to us, it's key to our survival, firing up quick, protective health and safety messages and prompting immediate, automatic fight, flight or freeze behaviours. Threat is not therefore the place of the calm, nuanced, cognitive functioning, story focus or memory that is needed to follow and enjoy a book.

Books also need us to use our imagination to empathize with others and to create and occupy worlds, but a threat imagination only takes apart and deconstructs.

But of course you're like this. We know that the depression demons have set up camp around the brain's judging panel and removed their ability to remember things, to make decisions and to process thoughts and emotions. They're just languishing around your hippocampus re-reading the entire works of Shakespeare and comparing notes, while the functions in your brain are trying to work out the difference between left and right. Of course reading is going to be difficult.

There's a lot of comfort to be found in re-reading a book

that you've loved already, just as I find there is comfort to be had in the sounds of a TV show or film that you pretty much know off by heart. Sometimes hearing the predictable comedy of Phoebe Buffay making fun of Ross Geller's dinosaur fossils can actually make you feel like you're not, in fact, totally alone in your darkness.

There's a bit of a concept that spending three hours with a TV show makes you less interesting and less intellectual than if you were to spend three hours with a book. Reading for an hour makes you bright and interesting. Watching TV for an hour makes you a lard-ass. Realistically, whatever keeps you happier and out of the gloom makes you smarter for choosing to do it in the first place. So well done, us, bring on the Netflix.

Sometimes the most blah, non-eventful television can be the most restorative. In this I'm including episodes of *Friends* you've seen countless times, endless seasons of *Gilmore Girls* in which only about two things happen during the entire span of the show, or something like a property development show if you can stomach five hours of Kirstie and Phil.

Comforting TV is calm, non-provoking and unchallenging. It's not anything that 'really makes you think, doesn't it?' and definitely has no cliffhangers or upcoming drama that could be ruined by a spoiler if you didn't watch it at the exact same time as the US release via some dodgy illegal streaming platform.

In fact, just today I was on the phone with Dré talking about all the joys of remortgaging the house that was bought together with hopes and dreams of love and joy, which we're now both moving out of because we've split up. The break-up, is, quite obviously, feeling hugely traumatic for both of us: it's sixteen years of life by each other's side suddenly stopping. We were together for more time than we weren't together, which is quite mad, considering that before we were sixteen we spent a good few years not being able to shit unsupervised.

Anyway, I was talking to Dré and mentioned to him casually that I had been rewatching *Friends* a lot, from the beginning. He hates *Friends* (not the reason we broke up – but it was a close call) but told me that he'd been staying up until the early hours rewatching, from the beginning, *Jonathan Creek*. Two perfect examples of fairly inconsequential television acting as a comfort blanket during times of bleak, bleak misery. Hurrah for Caroline Quentin.

However, there are some people who believe so fully in the power of a transformative film – including that a film can actually be transformative in the first place – that they now prescribe 'cinema therapy' as an accompaniment to their counselling.

The concept behind movie therapy is simple: by watching the relationships between characters, the issues they deal with and how they tackle their problems, our emotions are heightened. Films encourage us to release our emotions, and when we choose films that can mirror our current situations, this emotional release will be all the more significant. As we're watching all the goings on as a third-party voyeur, we're not consciously putting our defences up so can, in theory, identify what's making us feel a certain way and perhaps recognize triggering situations.

There's also a wealth of research to suggest that watching sad films or TV shows actually makes us happier, as we're more likely to come away from the viewing thinking about what we've got that we're grateful for.

I guess it depends on the movie, but it certainly explains why *EastEnders* has had such a long shelf life.

When 'prescribed' a film, patients or clients must watch it a few times to fully 'digest the therapeutic benefits'. I've never had cinema therapy myself but am skeptical of the practice. Surely if a therapist can recognize that you'd relate to a particular character, or find some answers in a particular plot, they could, well, just tell you? Also, it seems like a big ask for a therapist to also have a full working knowledge of every film ever made. Just saying.

But apparently it works. Films are made to have mass appeal and be comprehensible even though sometimes complex. Being told 'Ah, I see, you're just like Maleficent, the mistress of all evil' might not be totally well received, but watching the film and figuring out that you relate to the child-hating woman who was wronged by her former lover and now lives alone while cursing the local infants... it would make more sense, I guess. Also, relating to a film character's struggle does make it easier to explain yours to someone else, as you could just get them to watch the film.

It's an odd one, cinema therapy. I can see how it would perhaps be a good side dish to counselling, but to me, it doesn't stand up enough on its own to be a whole therapeutic concept. As in, I'm not entirely convinced it's 'a thing' that's not just the regular practice of watching films. You don't need to be depressed to be able to apply film scenes to your own life. If you're seriously struggling with depression and suicidal thoughts, you probably won't be impressed with hearing that you could make great progress out of your misery if you would only just sit down and watch *The Jungle Book*. It sits in the same bucket as retail therapy: proven to help when done right, but you don't necessarily need a therapist to tell you to do it.

If you can concentrate on reading, then I really would suggest consuming some fiction to give your mind a break from your demons. There are plenty of books (suggested previously) about depression that certainly made me feel more understood, and like I had a friend going through a similar experience. Don't put too much pressure on yourself to read tonnes of books – or even chapters. Focus on a specific segment or two and try to absorb it, if reading anything more seems like way too much.

The clapbacks

Isn't it obvious? It's this book, innit.

CHAPTER 15

... you should have said something

We're all talking about mental health a lot more now than we were ten years ago, which is great... isn't it? I think it is, but at the same time 'being part of the conversation' sounds like something I absolutely do not want to do.

I don't really want to post a selfie with an #invisibleillness tag across it (and, as we know, depression can be quite visible indeed). I don't want to introduce myself to a group of people and tell them all how long I've been feeling bleak for as they tilt their heads sympathetically and nod along. I honestly don't want to constantly explain what it's like to have depression, as I'm utterly convinced that everyone has it anyway and I'm just being a condescending tit, and I don't want to make an announcement across my open-plan office that states, 'Hey, I've got depression and I'M NOT AFRAID!'

Depression removes fear anyway. The more realistic announcement would be, 'I've got depression and I don't give a flying fuck what happens in this office or to me or my career and I hope I get run over on the way home,' but that's not what 'the conversation' is meant to be about, is it?

There are adverts, posters and slogans seemingly everywhere telling us that getting help for depression can be 'as easy as just telling someone' – which makes me want to throat-punch whoever came up with it. In the aftermath of suicides, people all over the internet post declarations of help being available. 'You are not alone, someone cares,' they say. 'Just reach out.'

It's not as easy as that, though, is it? A few months before Caroline Flack killed herself, she posted on her Instagram account that she'd tried to reach out to a friend for help and support, and they'd told her that they'd found her to be 'draining'. That's enough to make you never want to share any of your thoughts ever again.

Telling someone that you're depressed still feels like you're making everyone suspicious of you. It feels like they think you're weak, like you've tricked them all, and like they might never trust you or want to see you ever again.

Also, the actual 'getting help' part can be much more difficult than just 'reaching out'. Earlier I mentioned my friend who couldn't get a doctor's appointment for months, and he's of course far from the only one in that situation. The waiting lists for therapy, medications, GP appointments and referrals are longer than *War and Peace*, and the hospitals and surgeries are straining with too many patients and not enough funding to cope. It's not the doctors' fault. The system is orchestrated in a way that makes things easy to miss, easy to forget or easy to just not be recorded properly. I won't be surprised if the NHS has been privatized by the time you're reading this, and getting a doctor's appointment now costs £50 on top of the six-week waiting time.

At the time of writing, patient notes in hospitals are still mostly handwritten, and some doctors can have up to fifteen logins for different parts of the NHS technology and record systems; a different username and password for X-rays, for test reports, for rotas – for everything.[54] Currently, all the patient record systems are linked in Wales, but most hospitals in England have their own separate systems, which are all totally unlinked. This is undoubtedly making a huge contribution to the 'slipping through the net' that can happen, and won't help cases of patients being released from psychiatric wards only to then end up on a five-month waiting list for therapy that will help them through recovery.

'Getting help' is not that simple, but thanks for the 'motivational' poster.

Look, I get it that I am part of 'the conversation' by writing a whole book about crappy mental health, but the book, rambling as it is, has hopefully helped explain to those not in the know that depression is way more complex than you ever thought it could be. Hopefully it has also helped reassure those with depression that they're not the only mad person in town, and that although it's different for everyone there's probably someone else somewhere who's had the same frightening thoughts as you have, or who's felt the same gut-wrenching feelings. Sometimes the feelings are so numbing that there's no way to describe or explain how you're feeling, because really you're just feeling nothing.

Telling a friend or loved one that you're depressed seems intimidating and pointless before you actually do it. For starters, the word 'depressed' just does not do justice to the physical aching and heaviness, the cloudy fog in your brain and the perpetual and permanent state of misery you've found yourself in. For the main course (I write this hungry), what the hell are they supposed to do about it once you've told them? They've probably got their own issues, how the hell are they meant to navigate yours? And finally, the icing on the cake, the question on everybody's lips that nobody ever asks because we're all convinced that we know the answer: why would they even care?

For me, this is why talking therapy was such a life changer – and I swear I'm not being a hyperbolic vapid millennial when I say that. It changed and may have even saved my life. Talking about how you feel to someone who is literally paid to listen to you and who you never have to see outside of those conversations, to me, was perfect. Eventually.

Talking therapy (often called counselling) worked well for me because I could tell somebody all my darkest thoughts without the worry of horrifying them and inflicting them with constant concern or worry about me, which most probably would have happened if I'd tried to have the same conversations with my family or friends. It's not that I don't trust my loved ones, it's more that I don't want to burden them with my mental health or change their behaviour or approach to me.

There are a few talking therapy options available, including the cognitive behavioural therapy we talked about earlier in this book. They include:

- **Cognitive behavioural therapy (CBT):** This is very practical therapy that aims to change your behavioural patterns as a result of really examining how you react to and think about your life. It usually involves drawing charts of thoughts or drawing circles around things, and there are a lot of resources online you can start looking into before you tackle it with a therapist. A CBT practitioner can help you identify false or unhealthy thoughts, and train your brain into replacing them with positive, healthy thoughts instead.

- **Dialectical behaviour therapy (DBT):** Similar to CBT but adapted for those of us who experience emotions really intensely. It's still centred around learning behavioural change, but also self-acceptance. It was established to help treat borderline personality disorder (BPD) and is now used to help people with suicidal thoughts and extremely unstable emotions. I didn't actually know that this existed before double checking my research for this book. It sounds pretty good.

- **Eye movement desensitization and reprocessing (EMDR):** Emma the nurse told us about her experience applying for this, earlier in the book. It's a talking therapy that was developed to help people with post-traumatic stress disorder (PTSD) and helps the brain 'reprocess' traumatic memories so that the patient can acknowledge them, accept them and work through them. As it involves revisiting painful moments, it's really important to have a good network of supportive folk around you who know what you're going through in therapy.

- **Counselling:** This is the more 'traditional' therapy that you will have seen in film and TV. From my experience there is never the chaise longue that I imagined laying back dramatically upon while pouring out my worries, but a kind therapist who helps you recognize and work through knots and difficulties in your life. Counselling for depression was really effective for me when I stopped labelling it as a 'lame American trope of BS'.

When I could bring myself to register on the Mind.org website, let alone leave the house and go to an initial session, I expected my therapist to fix me in the first go. Medication alone hadn't 'cured' me (but I'm sure contributed to the fact that I was motivated to seek further help) so I thought it was perhaps something about me as a person that wasn't working.

I sat in front of this calm, kind woman and sobbed for an hour, trying to articulate how horrific I felt. I said that, yes, I do have suicidal thoughts all the time, and then carried on sobbing, doing that lush sniffly hiccup thing you do when you're incompetently trying to stop.

After blubbing in a chair for an hour (fifty-five minutes if you want to be pedantic), I was then utterly dismayed when she didn't rise from her seat and pronounce, 'Well, it's clear that you're feeling this way because of this, so stop doing that and you'll be fine.'

What did I expect? We're living in an age of instant gratification; we have access to any song in the world in our ears, any cuisine in the world on our doorstep and any film in the world on our screens at the tap of a phone screen. We are the closest we've ever come to being Sabrina the Teenage Witch; if we press our phone three times, a pizza might arrive – or a taxi, a cleaner, a masseuse, or even someone to slather you with hot wax and rip out your pubes. Why couldn't a brain fix be the same?

I honestly expected her to say something like, 'Look in the mirror and repeat the following text, and during the night you shall levitate at midnight and tomorrow you shall awaken a new woman who will live forever in bliss.'

Despite the lack of instant gratification, I forced myself to return for another session. This time, the therapist managed to get another feeling out of me rather than just misery: rage. This was unexpected, but the majority of her questions in this session were about my immediate family and the relationships I've had and have with them. 'It's not about my family,' I told her, sternly (I thought). 'How I feel has absolutely nothing to do with my family. We have a great relationship – I was just sending a gif to the family WhatsApp group on the bus on the way here! CHANGE THE SUBJECT, FOR GOD'S SAKE.'

This was the third form of talking therapy that I'd tried after the disastrous bout of CBT. Finding a therapist is hard – and damn expensive. When putting my feelings into literal boxes and circles turned out to do absolutely diddly squat, I felt like I should at least try talking therapy, despite being still mostly convinced it was a load of needless American tripe. But for talking therapy to be effective you need to actually like your therapist – or at least respect them. My Goldilocks approach found me a great therapist eventually but it started off shakily.

My first visit to a therapist hadn't done much to quell the thought that therapy was all twoddle. After scrolling through Counselling Directory (an excellent resource for finding therapists if you're in the UK and can afford to see one) and after I made myself stop judging therapists on their choice of haircut, I settled on a new therapist, a local-ish lady who was very experienced.

Walking up the path to her front door in North London, I felt like a prize twat. 'What am I even doing here?' I thought to myself. 'I despise talking about my feelings, and the therapists on the telly all seem really, really annoying. Anyway, I'm only SAD. It's not like I've lost a limb while fighting to save the life of a child in a war and now have PTSD and an edgy limp.' If it wasn't for the cancellation policy meaning I would still have to pay if I didn't show up, I would have pulled a 180 in her front garden and walked away.

But, I was already there, and if I was going to set fire to sixty quid I might as well watch the flames dance. She buzzed me in (fancy) and I was taken to a soulless, grey-walled and carpeted room with two armchairs facing each other, two glasses of water on a tiny circular table in between them and a box of super-soft tissues on the side. Groan.

'Take a seat,' she said, gesturing to the chairs. We sat down and looked at each other. 'Tell me what made you book this appointment,' she asked.

'Because I'm depressed,' I replied monotonically. That's a fiver gone already.

'OK, let me tell you how I can help you,' she began, before reeling through her qualifications and experience while I sat there silently, thinking it was costing me over £1 a minute to hear her tell me what I'd already read online. 'So,' she sipped from her water and sat back in her chair, clasping her hands together. A disappointing sense of déja vu washed over me as she proceeded to look over her glasses and say, 'Tell me about your family.'

Another therapist asked me if I wanted children (spoiler: NOPE) before saying that my severe self-loathing is probably because I'm the eldest child, and when my little sister was born everyone praised everything she did while scolding me for learning to walk and walking into/picking up the wrong things. I don't even know if I *could* walk when my sister was born, but this notion just seemed ridiculously implausible to me. I was sick to the back teeth of therapists hammering me about my family, as if they were to blame.

Turns out the whole line of family questioning is actually

nothing to do with your therapist thinking that Philip Larkin was onto something, but instead about them finding out about your 'attachment style'. Your attachment style will have formed in your early childhood, based on how you interacted with caregivers. Attachment styles then come to fruition in adulthood, influencing how you select a romantic partner, how you conduct the relationship and how relationships tend to end. This 'relationship' can also transfer into relationships you have with your friends, your work life and, yes, your family.

The key thing is, though, that dysfunctional attachment styles can be changed, and this is often the basis of most therapy. This is why a lot of therapists will ask about your relationship with your family, even if you're coming to therapy with a predicament that doesn't involve your family at all and is instead way more about how you want to off yourself despite having loving parents and a best friend for a sister.

For example: people who grew up with an alcoholic parent will annoyingly find themselves swooning over partners who also drink a lot. Those of us who grew up with argumentative parents will find ourselves waiting for the accusatory text messages from partners who like to argue with us, too. PANIC NOT, you're not subconsciously trying to bonk your parents if you do this, you're actually trying to take control of a situation in which you felt helpless when you were a child. That sounds loads better. However, by trying to 'fix' the problems you had in childhood, you're actually re-opening the wounds and putting yourself in a vulnerable position where you'll likely end up feeling unloved. If you work through your feelings with a therapist, you'll find yourself becoming attracted to a different 'type' than you've become used to.

Yeah, I've read a lot of books about therapy. Soz. Just saving you the time.

My family has a history of depression. My grandma killed herself when she was in her fifties, and other family members are currently being visited by the demons, too. Even so, it took us years to start talking about it to each other. When we did, I found myself reacting in all the ways that I knew I shouldn't. When I heard about a loved one's darkest period, I instantly thought back to what I was doing at that time and how I could have been more loving and more supportive, and that I might have been able to keep them out of this depression if only I'd been better to them. Even though **I know this isn't true.**

I'd hate for anyone I love to be thinking that about me. Even the thought of it makes me crumble.

I know depression is a medical illness and it can't be 'loved out of you', but at the same time, I do think love can prevent you from suicide (up to a certain point, at least). It certainly has for me.

There is a lot that the depression demons do to convince you that nobody loves you, or even cares about you a little bit. Most of the illness convinces you that, actually, everyone would be better off without you – if they even notice at all that you're gone. It's not about you thinking that you'd rather die than spend another moment with your friend Jenny, but about a yearning to just not be alive anymore. To just stop. To just stop this living and throbbing and exhaustion and pain and to just be nothing.

In Matt Haig's book *Reasons to Stay Alive* he talks about the time when he walked to the edge of a cliff and almost kept on walking. He recalls wishing, as he stood on that cliff edge, that he didn't have a family or a girlfriend who loved him, because if he didn't then he'd be able to take the one more step needed to end it all.

It seems very 'after-school special' that the only thing that's scary when you're not afraid of death is love. When you're really, genuinely not afraid of dying, the only thing that can bring any amount of real concern into your life is the thought of the people you love dying.

But… would it also be a release, and permission for you?

I am about to share my Darkest Ever Thought, which no longer troubles me with its presence but certainly used to. I'm scared to share it, but how can we make progress if we still keep secrets?

Deep breath. The thought was that when my family dies, I will obviously be crippled with pain, of course, but also it would mean that I could then die, too, because they wouldn't be left behind and blaming themselves. I'll admit in my darker times my mind has travelled to the regions of 'what if they all died in an accident, and it was painless and not scary for them? Then I could die too and it would all be over.'

I don't feel like that anymore. I'm actively working on separating this illness from myself and on being involved in a good life.

However, sometimes, in specific circumstances, when people kill themselves there's a small part of me that's a little bit happy for them having found their release and ended their suffering. Am I the only one? Is that an awful thing to say? I don't know anymore.

Yes, it's debilitating knowing that someone else has felt as dark as you have, knowing that they've had the hollow void of feeling apart from a hot pain of stabbing misery. It's a throat-punch of awful realization that this person has felt so unbearably, desperately miserable that they wanted to stop it all and could see no other way out of the pain. A feeling that you, too, know only too well.

But... but. But sometimes, in very particular cases, I do feel relieved for them. They managed to make it stop. They're not living in pain anymore and they're not waking up every day wishing that they hadn't. They're not waking up. They won. They took control and stopped the pain. They got what they wanted.

I must clarify here that this school of thought doesn't apply when I hear about people who have died by suicide after living a much-scrutinized life in the public eye, under the microscope of the media lens, or where a third party was clearly hugely contributary towards their decision to take their own life – if they were abused, for example. Most of us will never know what was really going through the mind of anyone who kills themselves, but it's undeniable that the media today hounds people (women in particular) with an unrelenting spite and venom. It's undeniable that this hugely contributes to a state of poor mental health.

Look at how the media toxically point fingers at Meghan Markle. Look at what they wrote about Amy Winehouse. About Princess Diana. About Caroline Flack. In instances like this there is no part of me that will ever feel remotely glad for those who have killed themselves following the brutality of bullying – famous or not. Nobody deserves to be targeted and attacked to the extent that they end their own life to make it stop.

Depression and suicidal thoughts can come from so many things, and we know that everyone who suffers is going through a totally different struggle to anyone else. A lot of people have depression that has a 'cause', i.e. it came from an event or experience, like the loss of a loved one or poisonous bullying.

Then there are those who have depression for seemingly no reason at all. There's nothing 'to complain about' or nothing going horrifically wrong, yet they find themselves utterly, unbearably miserable. These are the people who make me feel partly, smidgenly glad for them; there was no getting out of misery, so they got out of life to end it. They're not hurting anymore and they took control. I respect that.

'What the actual FUCK are you talking about?' was the response I got when I once shared this sentiment. 'No! No, no, no! This isn't what you're supposed to think! What the... how can you think that?'

OK, so maybe not *quite* everyone else is depressed, too.

Of course, this kind of response to those types of thoughts is, as much as you can say, 'normal'. But it's this kind of response that puts people off telling their trusted or loved friends how much pain they are truly feeling. It's a sharp reaction of 'Oh my shit, what is going on in Kate's head? I never knew she was mad!' and a reminder that, actually, there's probably something seriously quite wrong with you. Then there's the fact that this person will probably now tiptoe around you, constantly ask if you're OK and be worried that you're going to kill yourself while they nip to the loo.

So we don't tell people.

But I know I should. We all know we should, but it's all so overwhelming and consuming and giant that putting it into words seems like a Herculean challenge, so we just say, 'I'm not feeling too great', 'I'm not feeling very well', or if we're really brave, 'I've been feeling a bit down' – which is the most honest, and yet the one most usually met with, 'Ahhh cheer up, it's meant to be hot tomorrow!'

When my friend killed himself it was 32°C and sunny.

The lack of understanding of mental illness is what shuts the doors for us. That, teamed with the terrifying premonition that if you do confide in someone they'll always tilt their head to one side and soften their voice as they ask, 'But how are you really feeling in yourself?' forevermore.

When people say that their depressed friends can talk to them, they don't know that a lot of what their friend really wants to say is likely that they would rather be dead so that they don't feel so awful anymore, because they can't see how anything else would change it. It's not helpful to say this to someone, but when it's the only thought swelling up inside you it's also unavoidable. What is someone supposed to respond with? All the 'things will get better' and 'you have so much to live for' attempts fall on deaf ears. They do not have anything to live for, as far as they're concerned, because living is fucking painful. Every day it's painful. It physically hurts, everywhere, and it would be a lot easier to just bow out of life and not have anyone make a big deal about it.

But I will say this: when I told Dré I was depressed, my behaviour 'clicked' for him. So, while it might not hugely help *us* out if we talk about it, there's a strong chance it will crucially help out someone you love. My 'revelation' of depression made Dré realize that actually he wasn't pissing me off all the time. I wasn't avoiding him constantly and hiding in a dark bedroom to run my side-job as a voice on an erotic phoneline OR because I couldn't stand to speak to him or look at his lovely face. I was depressed. It all made sense.

It's almost funny (almost) that as someone with such a deep understanding of what it's like to be depressed (in my own way), I find it a huge struggle to know what to say to someone in a similar position. All I want to say is, 'Yeah, I know, it's fucking shit, isn't it? Let's lie in the dark and cry,' but that's not really advised or productive.

A friend once called me when he was feeling unfathomably dark. He had lost all hope, he didn't see the point in going on anymore and wanted to be stopped from 'doing something stupid'. I headed over to see him immediately, but en route wondered to myself, 'Wait a minute, what do I actually have to say to him that's gonna make him stop?'

What I found actually helped him was for me not to talk at all, really, but to listen. I sat down in front of him and just said, 'Tell me,' and he did. I tried to remember the behaviour of Therapists I Have Known, and asked him things like where he thinks those feelings are coming from. I didn't tell him what to do, and acknowledged that yeah, life's a shitshow, and I'm here if you wanna talk about it.

Nothing evangelical, but it seemed to work, and I think if I was talking to someone about it, that's how I'd like them to respond, too.

When people kill themselves, those who are left behind are shrouded in guilt. They're filled up with it, like they've had a guilt-injection and it's spread through every vein and millimetre of their body. They wonder if their friend had been trying to tell them, and they'd not realized or even chosen not to hear it. They repeat details over and over and convince themselves that if they'd only said this thing on that day instead of doing that other thing, their friend might still be here.

'But why didn't they say something?' they'll wonder. 'Why didn't they just tell me how they were feeling? I could have helped!'

Could you, though?

Having been a sad sack for years, I've spent a lot of time reading about other people being sad sacks. For years I've been trying to educate myself about the options and treatments and potential methods of recovery for sad sacks around the world, I'm honestly not sure if anyone can fix us forever. If any*thing* can fix us forever. Although, as I hope you've discovered in these pages, there are a lot of things that can help make us feel more in control and make the illness more separate and manageable.

Exercise certainly helps, baths are nice and washing yourself is a good thing to do. Eating well is a good idea and there are medications and therapy options that can help us, sure, but they don't actually make it all go away, do they?

Will it ever go away, or can we just throw all our efforts at the demons to fend them off and shrink them down, and as long as we keep throwing exercise, therapy and orgasms at them, they'll never grow back into their previous, fully monstrous form?

Sure, people can support us and even though our faces don't have expressions and our bodies don't seem capable of emotional responses, my God are we grateful for even the tiniest support. The tiniest gesture, the effort not to push a line of 'how are you?' questioning or to just show up... thank you. But the only person who can help you is yourself.

The clapbacks

When someone tells you 'you should have said something' it can also have the fun effect of making you feel guilty, or like you have offended this person by not talking about your depression to them. Perhaps the following could help:

'It's hard for me to talk about it because I don't fully understand it myself. Thanks for the support, though. Chances are I won't let you know if I need anything, because I don't know what I need. I'm trying to pay attention to myself so I can care for myself, but for now I just need your friendship and for you not to treat me any differently. I might decline events a lot, but I'd love to keep being invited. It means a lot to know you're thinking of me.'

CHAPTER 16

Why don't you have a holiday, sweetheart?

This one is probably the least offensive of the lot, I think, because a change of scenery and getting outdoors really, really does help – if you can manage to bring yourself to do it in the first place. Now, a seven-day all-inclusive trip to Magaluf might not be quite the type of trip to heal you forever and leave you a refreshed, radiant new beacon of joy, but getting away from your regular life can give you a much-needed different perspective.

When I was working at *Cosmo* and was frying my brain and my liver constantly and aggressively, I knew I needed to do something dramatic and that it probably shouldn't be killing myself. I was staying out drinking until the wee hours and then waking up to get into work early to get a head start, almost in an attempt to just feel something other than numbness. I took on extra work as a way to be distracted from the demons, and when I left the company they advertised for three different jobs to cover the work I had been doing. This isn't me being smug, this is me reflecting on being DUMB. Whatever you allow to happen will always continue, and I allowed the extra work to come in and I worked extra hours to make it all go smoothly, before going out to put some extra hours in at the bars afterwards.

I wasn't so much burning the candle at both ends as I was dousing myself in cheap tequila and just setting myself on fire.

So I quit. I booked a four-month trip to Central America, the Philippines and Indonesia, and told my bosses I was leaving this job to go to Mexico. It felt like a physical weight had been taken off my chest. I just had the three-month notice period to finish first…

In a surprise turn of events, it seemed to really piss a lot of people off when they learned that I had voluntarily left my 'great, glamorous job' to travel. Lots of people also enjoyed poking fun at the *Eat Pray Love* direction I was choosing, and I had a few well-wishers and hopes that I would 'find myself' once away. Ha. I've already found myself, darling, and I hate her. I'm going away to lose myself completely and maybe see a cool fish. Jumping off what many saw as 'my career ladder' and jacking it all in was the best thing I've ever done.

Of course, 'jacking it all in' sounds pretty breezy, when in fact I had some very hard work to do financially. Having no children (thank God) or other dependants to care for, I was in the privileged position to be able to spend my income on myself. So, as soon as I'd planned to go away, I started putting a third of my wages (after rent) into a savings account.

The little money that I saved wasn't enough to get me very far in London, but in the countries I was desperate to visit fifty quid would sort out a few nights' accommodation. Disclaimer: I also got a credit card. I figured I'd pay the minimum off while I was away, and would rather be poor when I got back home than be restricted in beautiful countries abroad.

As someone who was attached to a brand in every job and attached to a boyfriend for sixteen years, I was finding myself constantly referred to as 'Kate from *Cosmo*', or 'Kate and Dré' and was utterly convinced I wouldn't be worth anything without the crutch of a 'cool' job or a wonderful partner who everybody loves.

This trip was planned to remove myself as far from my normal life as possible, so Central America seemed like a good place to start. I was intrigued by the varied weather, wildlife, currencies, and a lot of still-developing countries practising traditional ways of life, like Guatemala, where most of the women still wear traditional Guatemalan traje attire (contrasted with most of the men wearing jeans and sports jackets).

Once the plan was in my head, it was excruciating to keep getting the Tube every day and going to work, but I actually found huge solace in changing all my passwords to FUCKTHISYAYMEXICO and suggest anyone else in limbo does the same. Even if you're just planning a weekend trip somewhere, or a visit to a friend for an evening, changing your passwords that you have to use every day really does help to remind you that there are hopefully better times a-coming.

Working out my notice was tedious, but it was speckled with visits to STA Travel to try to find the cheapest possible route for my journey; because I'm demanding and didn't know when I'd get the chance to visit my fuckit-list countries again, this included a (regretful) thirty-hour trip from Mexico City to Manila, via LA and Hong Kong – and that was the mid-range price, the dirt-cheapest would have taken seventy-two hours. Hard nope to that.

Saving up enough money to book the ticket in the first place gave me an injection of empowerment (I know, I sound like

Oprah) and made me feel like I'd taken control. I HAD taken control, I was actively trying to get away from my daily life, which I was busy hating, and running away to Mexico seemed like the answer. I was being utterly selfish and doing something just for me, abandoning everything I hated at home and truly fucking off for a while. The confirmation screen assuring me that the plane ticket was booked gave me a jolt of joy I hadn't felt since I accidentally sat on my phone when it was on vibrate.

The part of the screen that showed me how much money I'd just spent didn't inflict quite such a joyful response.

I changed my desktop background to be a regular rotation of beaches I wanted to visit, and was incessantly reading about routes and guides to remote villages while booking the most obscure, serene, secluded accommodation I could find. I wanted out of the London cattle market and into a Mexican jungle.

Getting involved in researching the areas I wanted to visit, booking hostels in advance for the busy dates (I was going to be away for Christmas and New Year's Eve and I may be a depressed buffoon, but I know how accommodation books up, OK?) and watching documentaries about the archipelagos I would be visiting was also a magnificent way to take my foot off the gas at work. Well, that and the fact that I'd decided I was leaving anyway, so I didn't need to care as much.

We didn't really need a professional study to tell us that anticipating something great will increase our happiness, but some people did one anyway and it also showed that anticipating experiences makes us happier than anticipating material/tangible purchases.[55] Even shoes.

I was tits-deep in Attenborough documentaries at the time (also a very soothing TV recommendation for when you're feeling shit, but depending on what state you're in there's a strong chance you'll cry about a polar bear) and desperate to see the Galapagos, so that was my first stop, via Quito. You can't just rock up to the Galapagos and go iguana-watching, though, you have to go on a group trip because it's such a protected national park, so I went through a tour company and booked a camping trip with a group of strangers. Gross.

Eating a 'last British meal' of fish and chips at Heathrow, I still felt exactly the same. Of course. Going through security at Terminal 5 doesn't really do much to kickstart a journey of emotional release.

Sitting on a hard bed in a threadbare room in Ecuador, feeling that bizarre over-tired-yet-a-bit-loopy jet lag feeling, I wondered what the hell I was doing. I was SO far away from anyone I knew, and suddenly this felt like the most counterproductive idea I'd ever had; what would make me feel better without all the distractions of work and friends and all the bars in Soho to occupy my brain? Now I was just the same sad twat, but in Ecuador. It was *Sad Twats Abroad*, series one.

I decided to go for a walk to get my bearings of the area – but I wasn't allowed. 'No, ma'am, we don't let women go out alone here after 10 p.m.,' the receptionist told me. 'It's very dangerous.' So that was that. I went back upstairs, had a little cry and deleted every social media app from my phone so that I couldn't see all the cosy wintery things my friends were doing. If I was going to do this alone, I was going to do this alone.

Well, as alone as you can be on a group camping trip.

Thankfully I was in super-solitude mode when I had booked this first part of the trip, and had plumped for the slightly more expensive (but dear God, so worth it) 'single camper' package, rather than sleeping half an inch away from a stranger's face in the damp. Nice one, past Kate.

The next morning, the group all met downstairs in the hotel. God, these people were perky. Some of them were on the final week of a two-month trip up from the bottom of South America and had been on *a guided group trip the entire time* and all seemed very jolly hockey sticks and in-jokes and rah-rah-rah. Some of them were on their honeymoon. Some of them seemed like they'd intended to book that all-inclusive week in Magaluf but somehow ended up here (to further prove that point, those same people ended up asking our tour guide where there was a good nightclub. In the Galapagos. In Darwin's home of understanding evolution. In a protected, cherished, wildlife paradise. They wanted a bloody Jäegerbomb).

But the beauty of travelling alone is that you really can choose just how alone you want to be, and when. When I was on the Galapagos trip and then for the following few months when I was going solo, one of the best parts of the whole thing (apart from seeing the world 'n' all that) was that I was able to always choose if I wanted company or not. Staying in hostels meant there was generally some kind of bar crawl/free breakfast situation that would bring everyone together, and if I wanted company that day I'd go and join in. More often, though, I was just a loner and I fucking loved it.

So, it's the first night of our Galapagos adventure, and the group have all gone to bed in their tents (at about 8 p.m. due to the total darkness, a 4 a.m. start the next day and a distinct lack of nightclubs). Lying in my leaky tent, my cheeks getting intermittently splashed with cold dollops of rain water, I could hear the wind whipping through the trees next to me, and I thought 'It's going to be OK, actually.' If anything, every shitty hostel I was about to stay in for the rest of the trip would seem like the actual Ritz in comparison to a tent that rained on the inside, and in the morning I'd be out there in the Galapagos Islands. Thousands of miles away from the life that was making me sick.

But I was feeling a bit sick. Not the usual nausea that I felt, but a more targeted sickness, and a crushing weight of pain in my abdomen. Ooh, was I dying from a tropical disease? Cool.

Then I got my period. In the night. In the rainforest. In a tent that was raining on the inside.

Maybe an as-yet-undiscovered Galapagaen bear would smell the blood and come and devour me in my sleep, I wondered. It would be a shame as I wouldn't have had the chance to see the birds with blue feet from the documentaries, but at least it would be the end.

So you can be away from your stresses and on a beautiful tropical island in paradise (well, in a wet tent, but still in paradise) and still welcome a bear attack over another day.

The next day came (obviously, I'm not writing this from beyond the grave) and I will say, though, that the morning's boat ride and the feeling of the salty spray of the sea slapping me in the face, whipping through the tropical winds while I sat on the side of a speedboat, ripping through clear bathwater and past endless palm trees... well, that was starting to feel like a pretty good tonic for despair.

The scenery was undoubtedly helpful to my mental state. Everywhere was stunning and made me want to be constantly outside and staring at it. Being indoors felt like I was wasting it. Like someone else might use up all the staring and I'd miss it all. I was still depressed, yes, but I was depressed on a beach instead of on the Piccadilly Line. The people-less jungles, the infinite powder-blue sea, the towering volcanoes around deep-blue lakes… they all made my other life feel like just that. Another life.

There was also a feeling of accomplishment every time I managed to get the correct bus from a maze of a station in Costa Rica, or every time I managed to have a successful chat with someone in crappy Spanish, or every time I arrived at a hostel and was shown to my room and I thought, 'Hey, that worked.' When you constantly feel like a failure and you're slumping around with an inexplicable sense of guilt, and an inescapable feeling that you're letting everyone down, the joy of receiving the exact sandwich you hoped you'd ordered in a foreign language is not to be dismissed.

As well as the staggering natural scenery and the tiny joys of booking a bus ticket, there are the locals. Being immersed in a different way of living, in a culture with very different priorities and values to the culture you're used to, can actually make you appreciate other people. I know. So weird.

Speaking to local people and staying with local families, seeing an (often much simpler) approach to life so removed from what my 'normal' was, really made me think about what I wanted my 'normal' to be. I'm not saying it's a way of 'getting some perspective on your depression' because it's entirely possible to be aware of and see people living a difficult life, people struggling for food and finances, and still be depressed. Your depression will not disappear when you see people who are not as privileged as you are, but your brain will take into account the new experiences you're creating for yourself, and make more connections around the demons to help them shrink a little.

Every time we do something for the first time, we make a new connection in our brain. Exercising our brains by challenging ourselves and having new experiences will keep our brain flexible. A flexible brain with top-notch neuroplasticity is what we're all capable of having, and is just what a depressed demon-hoarder will need to be able to keep the demons at bay. The new stuff doesn't have to be a trip to Ecuador, it can be as little as a new route home from work, a new book or new music. It's basically just not getting stuck in your ways like a nanna.

The break from work also gave me a chance to do what all those mindfulness gurus are always wanging on about, and actually live in the moment. Escaping to a place you've never been to before – even if it's in your home country but totally removed from your everyday life – forces you to be more aware of your surroundings. You do look up and wonder if that magnificently coloured tropical bird is going to crap on you. You do take time to appreciate the feeling of whatever weather has been chucked at you, and you do start to notice things that might even go as far as making you think, 'Ooh, isn't that nice?'

Mindfulness. It actually happened. Woah.

Of course, as well as the giant tortoises and quetzals, I did have to encounter some other actual humans. Gross. Naturally, I met a lot of twats, but also lucked out a few times and found people who made me laugh, which (I think) is really all that matters on a trek like this. It's largely what matters most in life, isn't it? Laughing. If you're not laughing, then what's the point? If you feel like there is no point left, then you might as well laugh about it? Right?

Anyway, I met some people who were fun and clever and different, and who were all 'solo travellers', too, which made me feel like we had some natural sappy connection of shared desires or something. It was coming up to the end of December, and we travelled together for two great weeks. As it was Christmas, we botched together a very haphazard Secret Santa, and that Secret Santa over a very unfestive meal in Mexico was the source of the most validation I've ever had.

We were exchanging gifts wrapped in newspapers or train tickets or whatever else we had, and someone correctly guessed that a gift was from me. 'How did you know?' I asked him. 'Easy, mate,' he said. 'It was hilarious and took the absolute piss out of me, but was also really, really thoughtful.' Thank you, lovely Tom from Australia, who told me I had personality traits I never thought I would have. These were the words I didn't know I was so desperate to hear: validation outside of a job or a relationship. Growth.

Then that night I got super-drunk and lost my debit card, so it was hardly a spiritual transformation.

'Just quit your job and travel!' is truly crappy advice; the Instagram posters should really say, 'Work really hard, live like a pauper to save more money than you think you'll need, do your notice period, plan your finances and then have a short break to look at the trees and be nourished by the kindness of strangers,' but that's really not as catchy.

So yeah, travelling is lush. This much we know. It can distract you and soothe you and make you figure out what you prioritize. It won't cure your depression (will anything?) but it will make it more manageable and give your mind some peace.

Being on the other side of the world, in a different time zone from everyone that I knew, also surprised me by subconsciously making me realize who I wanted in my life and who I didn't. After a month of ten-hour bus journeys and only an hour or so where time zones overlapped and my friends and family in the

UK would be awake at the same time as me, I realized I'd both prioritized and forgotten about some pretty surprising people.

I found myself scrolling through my WhatsApps and realizing that there were some people I had not thought about for a single second since leaving. Truly out of sight, out of mind, but also out of inbox. Some of these people I used to see weekly when I was in London, or even work with. Turns out they must have been friendships of convenience or circumstance, as it seemed I didn't give a toss how they were doing, and they didn't give a toss about me. Excellent. Distance has a way of making you really think about your priorities.

It's probably important to say, though, that when I came back to London after my little trip, my depression felt more exacerbated than it had in a very long time. I felt like I was just going to have to slot back in to my 'old life' and carry on like before – and I was so miserable in the before. It was more than the 'post-holiday blues', though, when you feel like you're missing out on another life because you have to live this one.

Although, I really enjoyed an unexpectedly lusted-after M&S tuna and cucumber sandwich in Heathrow's arrivals area. It was lovely having a shower in a bathroom not used by fifty-seven people, and to put all my clothes in a washing machine that didn't make them smell burnt. It was refreshing to wake up without new mosquito bites or bits of my own skin flaking off. It was a stab in the chest to wake up in my old bedroom, though, as if nothing had happened.

How could everything seem the same when I felt like I had changed so much?

It was a numbness that came alongside thrumming anxiety. It was back to the insatiable tears. It was a claustrophobia but also a feeling of being lost. It was fucked.

I met up with friends and I felt entirely disconnected. I finally understood what people are harping on about when they refer to situations as being like 'an out-of-body experience, like you're watching yourself from above'. I didn't want to talk about my trip to anyone. I wanted to keep it all just for me. I felt an awful churn of anxiety, hollowness and sadness. I felt like a delinquent for wanting to be away again, when I'd thought I was really ready to come back home.

I felt so, so sad, and so uncomfortable. So out of place. So empty. So guilty for not appreciating my life of comparable luxury.

So I booked some more trips. I still had that credit card, so I chased the dragon with weekends in Europe and day trips to the coast. It felt like such a waste of time to stay in the same city for more than four days in a row, sinking back into the greyness and further away from the wind and space and sea.

Also, and this might sound insignificant, I bought a crap load of plants.

Nature is soothing to my depression, and even now that I'm not in an exotic country, getting outside and near some kind of greenery is a good way of not killing myself. It's one of the motivators that gets me to run (the five times a year I can manage it): seeing a new part of the world I haven't looked at yet. Combining the two, going on a trip somewhere and then having a run when you get there as a way of exploring what's waiting for you, seems to be a decent head-soother.

I worked freelance for a while, and saved up some money to go away for another month, this time to the South of France as it was a slightly more affordable plane fare. I moved on every few days, and I think that's really the key to feeling like you have some sort of purpose, some sort of reason to stay alive. Maybe? When you're travelling you are doing something; even if it's sitting on a bus where someone is selling fake passports to the passengers and being followed by three chickens, you're going. You're moving. You're doing. You feel purposeful and intentional and like you're not wasting your time being miserable. You're miserable, but on the way somewhere.

But of course, I'm not Beyoncé and I can't afford to go away all the time. So I took trips, I took short breaks, I filled my house with plants and tropical-looking wallpaper to try to invoke a feeling of being anywhere but North London, and then I left the country and moved to Paris.

Yeah, Paris isn't exactly known for its exotic climate, breathtaking underwater scenery and beautiful, unique vegetation – but it's a change and it's got wanky media jobs I can do so I can afford to live there. Three years after my quit-*Cosmo*-trip, and many other trips since, I decided to just ditch London altogether. OK, I might go back one day, but for now the plan is to stay away. Paris made sense as a starting point; French is sexy, croissants are medicinal and Paris has pretentious 'digital media content creator blah' companies I can fanny around in.

The UK is home to my greatest love story and subsequent big break-up. The most heart-shattering break-up with a man I will always love. It also offered me seemingly dull work opportunities with way too much corporate responsibility. Realizing that my mental health had pushed away the man who nobody will ever love as much as I do… I knew it was time to go. I didn't want to push anyone else away, and I didn't want to get stuck back into the tired trope of 'before', so I looked for jobs abroad, and applied for some in Paris. I got an interview, I got an offer and

I got on the Eurostar to go and live in a city where I don't know anyone and can't speak the language.

Très bon, then.

The move did have a bit of the desired effect, though, which was a surprise. Friends had warned that I might be putting too much expectation on moving away, and counting on 'when I get to Paris, everything will be different' too heavily.

I was more worried that if I was going to be living in a city where I didn't know a soul, what would there be to stop me descending further into darkness? There would be nobody to put on a pretence for, nobody who would know if I hadn't made it out of bed all day, and if I didn't turn up to work then *J'assume* I'd get a missed call from HR and that would be about it.

I was looking forward to the change of scenery and the influx of pastries, sure, but I was really concerned that this could go totally the wrong way and make my depression worse, as I'd have nobody to be accountable for.

To be honest, that part *has* kind of manifested. I don't have any reason to get up in the mornings if I'm not going to work, and often I do spend days feeling dark in the darkness. I don't have to come home from work and pretend that everything's OK, so the lows really can get very low.

But, weirdly, it means the achievements of actually going to work, or going outside, or washing or getting dressed or whatever, actually feel bigger. The accomplishments feel even more accomplished, because I've let myself get so much further down beforehand. I think feeling it, really, really feeling it, helps me a lot. Having a pretence and always trying to squash something away won't ever work in the long run, so letting it out is... a relief.

Turns out, being in a city where you know nobody really takes off a pressure that I didn't realize I was even carrying. Being somewhere that doesn't attach itself to any now-painful memories is easier to trudge around, and not speaking the language fluently makes it a lot easier to zone out from the noise.

Also, Paris is pretty and has shit loads of cheese.

I'm still depressed. Of course I'm still depressed, depression can't be poked out of you with a baguette, but I feel a bit more soothed. I think. It's hard to tell really, as going through what must be the world's most heart-shredding break-up in the history of all break-ups of all time (including Brad and Jen) has added another level of deep, deep sadness to me that wasn't there before. I didn't think I could get any sadder. LOL!

I'm still depressed, I'm just depressed in Paris. I still cry most days, but maybe now I cry with an alluring accent. I still have to leave work sometimes because my depression gets so heavy and oppressive that I can't hold myself together anymore, just now I cry my way home on le Metro, not le Tube.

I think a lot of the real reason behind moving somewhere where I knew no people and not many French words was about finding purpose. Something to do. A little goal to aim for. Learning French is really hard. Speaking French is even harder. It's a good distraction, and if I ever say something in French and a French person understands it then there's a teeny victory to be had. When that new colleague sent me a meme via Instagram DM I felt like I'd climbed Everest. Well, maybe Snowdonia.

Throughout this book I've been trying to reiterate that, yup, we're depressed, and, yup, it doesn't look like it's going away anytime soon, but – BUT – it might simmer down if we actually pay it some attention, stare it in the face and acknowledge its presence.

Being overtly aware that you're miserable sounds a bit dim – how could you not be aware? – but once you stop trying to ignore the misery and start actually factoring in its presence, you can start to try to manage it, or at least be prepared for it and try to work around it.

You might be depressed for the rest of your life – I truly believe that I will be – but know that the depression can blow in and out like rain clouds, or farts at a gig. Sometimes it's exceptionally windy (in all senses), and the storm will last for days. Weeks. Months. Years, sometimes. Sometimes, when we pay attention to the feeling in the air before the wind, we can prepare for the bad weather and it won't affect us so much. Sometimes the wind stops – but there's always a chance it could return.

Mental illness is probably always lurking, and it's up to us to know how to manage it. Nobody is going to come and save us.

This book isn't going to end with a cure for depression, a happy relationship, regular exercise and therapy and a glittering yacht sailing off into the sunset. Soz. It's ending with a relationship that broke down largely because of my brain breaking down. It's ending with me forcing myself to go to yoga when I feel wound up, and still always furiously hating the first fifteen minutes and talking myself into not stopping every single time. It's ending with me still regularly drinking too much, alone in my flat on a Tuesday night, just to get through the evening without thinking too much. It's ending with me still being fairly fucking miserable sometimes, but mostly knowing how to manage it.

The Big Dream is that this book is ending with you feeling more hopeful, too, or with more understanding or feeling like you're not the only one feeling the way you're feeling. I hope that you can use the lighter moments to plan for the darker moments, and get somewhere that feels more manageable and less of a doomy shitshow.

I'm trying to make mini plans to visit more of France on the weekends, both to unleash my crappy French on the innocent locals, but more to keep that feeling of travelling going. A feeling of moving, achieving and being outside with the pretty things. I know it will help me. I know it will.

The clapbacks

Honestly I really think this piece of unsolicited advice is a good one – it works for me, anyway, so here your priority is getting the person to pay for your trip, I think.

'That's a great idea, Jeff. I would if I could afford it, but I can't, so I'll probably die here... alone... miserable... on purpose... unless you've got any cash?'

Epilogue

While writing this book, I slipped back into some pretty heavy misery. That much may have been apparent during the quite frankly utterly joyful and uplifting reading, but there's certainly something about writing about a time when you found life to be meaningless that makes you think, 'Hey, wait a minute, life is still meaningless.'

This was punctuated by a failure to do or a re-instance of most of the themes of the chapter headings in this book. I fell out of exercise, because I was on a deadline. The news cycle continued to be a whirlwind of shite. I stopped reading. I had writer's block. I didn't want to get out of bed. I took days off work for depression again, and one day had to leave the office in the morning as I couldn't stop crying. I got thin. I got fat. I couldn't sleep. I slept too much.

I got signed off from work with depression after having a breakdown in a doctor's office when I went in with a cough. I wanted to get some proper medicine for it but ended up just crying and telling her how miserable I felt. It came out tumbling and stuttering and covered in snot and spit and other lush things doctors have to look at all day. She immediately wrote me off work for a week and told me to look after myself.

I think. It was in French.

She did ask if I had medication or a therapist, though. So that was nice.

'Right,' I told myself as I shuffled out of her office and back onto the Rue du le Croissant or wherever I was. 'This is fine. I'm writing a bloody BOOK about depression, I know how to take care of myself.' As I walked home I made lists in my head of what I was going to do to look after myself this week. It began with a big clean of the apartment, buying healthy food and teas, getting some fresh flowers, and – obviously – doing a face mask. I would go to some yoga classes nearby. Maybe I'll chance a run by the river. I know exactly how to keep the demons away because I am a Book Author and I Know Things.

When I got home, I opened the front door and went straight to bed. I stayed there for the next four months and nine hours, as the Covid-19 lockdown was announced that week.

We can wax lyrical about things that will help us, and we can laugh at how utterly crap everything is, if we're lucky. But it sometimes gets to a point when everything in your brain is asleep apart from the demons – please know that you're not alone in this. They're completely in control, they're swooping around your head and whispering to you in spits that you should die. You look around your flat to see what you have that could make that happen. You have quite a lot of things that would do the trick if you got really innovative. It's like a *Blue Peter* death special! You should have done this ages ago, the demons tell you.

You think of the people who you love.

You stay.

Notes and References

[1] https://www.who.int/news/item/02-03-2022-covid-19-pandemic-triggers-25-increase-in-prevalence-of-anxiety-and-depression-worldwide

[2] https://www.psychiatrictimes.com/view/post-covid-stress-disorder-emerging-consequence-global-pandemic

[3] https://www.nytimes.com/2022/05/13/business/great-resignation-jobs.html

[4] https://www.bupa.co.uk/newsroom/ourviews/anxiety-and-depression-the-link

[5] https://www.mayoclinic.org/diseases-conditions/depression/expert-answers/depression-and-anxiety/faq-20057989

[6] https://www.bupa.co.uk/newsroom/ourviews/anxiety-and-depression-the-link

[7] https://www.healthline.com/health/can-depression-make-you-sick#physical-symptoms

[8] https://www.sciencedaily.com/releases/2002/03/020311080611.htm

[9] https://www.ncbi.nlm.nih.gov/pmc/articles/PMC5144818/

[10] Daniel Levitin, *Successful Ageing: A Neuroscientist Explores the Power and Potential of Our Lives* (Penguin Random House USA, 2020), page 243

[11] https://www.kcl.ac.uk/ioppn/depts/pm/research/cfad/psilocybin-trials

[12] https://www.synthesisretreat.com/psilocybin-and-ssri-snri-interactions

[13] https://www.ncbi.nlm.nih.gov/pmc/articles/PMC6437683/

[14] https://www.rainbowrehab.com/executive-functioning/

[15] https://www.theguardian.com/society/2015/jun/30/chronic-depression-shrinks-brains-memories-and-emotions#maincontent

[16] https://www.ncbi.nlm.nih.gov/pmc/articles/PMC6437683/

[17] Florence Nightingale, *Notes on Nursing: What It Is, and What It Is Not* (Digireads.com, 2010)

[18] https://journals.plos.org/plosone/article?id=10.1371/journal.pone.0202246

[19] https://journals.sagepub.com/doi/10.1177/00139160121973115

[20] https://www.rsph.org.uk/about-us/news/instagram-ranked-worst-for-young-people-s-mental-health.html

[21] https://journals.plos.org/plosone/article?id=10.1371/journal.pone.0046362#s5

[22] https://www.health.com/condition/depression/multiple-social-media-sites-depression-anxiety

[23] https://www.bbc.com/future/article/20180928-the-surprising-truth-about-loneliness

[24] https://today.yougov.com/topics/lifestyle/articles-reports/2019/07/30/loneliness-friendship-new-friends-poll-survey

[25] https://www.ncbi.nlm.nih.gov/pmc/articles/PMC4045505/

[26] https://hbr.org/2017/04/a-face-to-face-request-is-34-times-more-successful-than-an-email

[27] https://www.npr.org/2017/06/04/531051473/the-millennial-obsession-with-self-care?t=1578513149102

[28] https://www.futurity.org/planning-hippocampus-brains-2007382/

[29] https://www.health.harvard.edu/blog/sad-depression-affects-ability-think-201605069551

[30] https://medicalxpress.com/news/2018-07-neural-link-depression-bad.html

[31] This is a good thing.

[32] https://www.mdmag.com/medical-news/patients-with-depression-show-increased-volume-left-hypothalamus

[33] https://www.researchgate.net/publication/230894480_Outpatient_Triple_Chronotherapy_for_Bipolar_Depression

[34] https://dsm.psychiatryonline.org/doi/abs/10.1176/appi.books.9780890425596.dsm04

[35] http://emilkirkegaard.dk/en/wp-content/uploads/The-great-comedians-Personality-and-other-factors.pdf

[36] https://www.ncbi.nlm.nih.gov/pmc/articles/PMC5702010/

[37] O'Connor L. E., Berry J. W., Lewis T. B., Stiver D. J., 'Empathy-based pathogenic guilt, pathological altruism, and psychopa-thology', *Pathological Altruism,* (eds) Oakley B., Knafo A., Madhavan G., Wilson D. S. (Cary, NC: Oxford University Press, 2012), 10–30.

[38] https://www.researchgate.net/publication/285296276_Empathy_and_depression_The_moral_system_on_overdrive

[39] https://hms.harvard.edu/sites/default/files/HMS_OTB_Spring10_Vol16_No2.pdf

[40] https://www.ncbi.nlm.nih.gov/pubmed/29215971

[41] https://www.telegraph.co.uk/news/2016/11/23/ice-cream-breakfast-makes-smarter-japanese-scientist-claims/

[42] https://www.psychologytoday.com/us/blog/brain-sense/201107/why-ice-cream-chases-the-blues-away

[43] https://www.psychologytoday.com/us/blog/the-antidepressant-diet/201008/serotonin-what-it-is-and-why-its-important-weight-loss

[44] https://pubmed.ncbi.nlm.nih.gov/6764927/

[45] https://www.beateatingdisorders.org.uk/types/orthorexia

[46] https://www.ncbi.nlm.nih.gov/pmc/articles/PMC4563885/

[47] https://foodandmoodcentre.com.au/smiles-trial/

[48] https://www.ncbi.nlm.nih.gov/pmc/articles/PMC3856388/

[49] https://www.ncbi.nlm.nih.gov/pmc/articles/PMC5133130/

[50] https://www.mentalhealth.org.uk/statistics/mental-health-statistics-suicide

[51] https://www.samaritans.org/about-samaritans/research-policy/suicide-facts-and-figures/

[52] https://www.mentalhealth.org.uk/news/survey-people-lived-experience-mental-health-problems-reveals-men-less-likely-seek-medical

[53] https://www.takingcharge.csh.umn.edu/reading-stress-relief

[54] https://www.bbc.co.uk/news/health-50972123

[55] https://journals.sagepub.com/doi/abs/10.1177/0956797614546556

Appendix

Resources for mental health support

GP: The first step should ideally be to **speak to your doctor** about how you're feeling. When I went, I self-diagnosed with an 'I think I'm depressed', which is fiiiiine, but it's more helpful to the doctor if you can describe how you're feeling and then they can diagnose you. They're the ones with the qualifications, after all. Don't worry about 'not being sad enough to get help', like I did – easier said than done, I know. Be honest about how you're feeling, and if you find it helpful to bring in some notes then do that.

Mind: Mind is the leading mental health charity in England and Wales and it's where I eventually found my Perfect Therapist Match. When I filled in a form online, I then booked an appointment over email. The first twenty-minute appointment is with a therapist who asks some initial questions so that you can be matched with another therapist most suited to you. I HATED the initial therapist dude, but loved the therapist I got matched with. Swings 'n' roundabouts, hey? Visit https://www.mind.org.uk/ or call 0300 123 3393. Email info@mind.org.uk or text 86463. They also have a lot of great information about supporting someone else who's struggling with their mental health.

Counselling Directory: Exactly what it says on the tin: a searchable directory of private counsellors. You can search by location, specialism and whether you'd like in-person or online appointments. The range of specialists is truly vast and doesn't just cover depression and anxiety. Visit https://www.counselling-directory.org.uk/ to have a gander.

Kate Mason: I leaned on Kate's wisdom and advice for a lot of this book. She was quoted throughout and really knows her stuff. Kate worked in the NHS for fifteen years before founding the Roots Psychology Group, a team of clinical psychologists, which you can find out more about at https://www.rootspsychologygroup.co.uk/ or by emailing kate@rootspsychologygroup.co.uk

Peter Klein: Another counsellor quoted heavily in this book, Peter specializes in treating problems such as stress, worry, anxiety, psychosis, depression and OCD with an emphasis on cognitive behavioural therapy. Visit https://www.counselling-directory.org.uk/counsellors/peter-klein

The Samaritans: Confidential support 24/7 with their free helpline, call 116 123.

Mental health support aimed specifically at men

The Lions Barber Collective: I just fucking love this initiative. This barber collective has trained its barbers in mental health support. They've not turned the barbers into qualified counsellors but provided a safe space to open up and be truly heard, while helped to access more support. They know it's OK to not be OK, and have rolled out this initiative nationwide. Visit https://www.thelionsbarbercollective.com/ or search 'locate a lion' to find a BarberTalk spot near you.

Men's Minds Matter: Focusing on depression, anger and rage, stress, anxiety and suicidal thoughts in men. Provides heaps of advice and resources at https://www.mensmindsmatter.org/

CALM: The Campaign Against Living Miserably provides support over webchat after 5 p.m. every day at https://www.thecalmzone.net/

Acknowledgements

After I wrote this book I spent many of the night's torturous small hours laying in bed and freaking out, asking myself why the fuckerydoo I had written this personal look into my brain. Even if nobody reads it apart from my family, *my family will read it* (so they tell me, anyway) *and they might be upset because it gets a bit dark and oh God what am I doing should I just pull out and say the publishers decided it was crap?* But pulling out (not like that) is part of 'the mental health problem', and I hope that whoever has read this has been able to see that depression absolutely isn't a choice. For me, it was nobody's fault. There is nobody to blame. It's an illness, and I've been pretty damn ill with it at times but am so much brighter and better now. There is a light somewhere. So thank you firstly to my family: Alice, Minnie and Stephen, for supporting me when I said I was 'gonna write a book about being glum' and for not getting too annoyed when I made HILARIOUS jokes about them all featuring in a non-existent chapter called IT'S ALL BECAUSE OF YOU. It's not because of you, obvs, and you all make my life so much richer and full of love, and I'm ridiculously glad to have you all and I love you so much.

The book wouldn't exist, though, if Jane Graham Maw hadn't seen potential in my 'doom and gloom' proposal and chapter ideas. Thank you, Jane, for persevering with the publisher hunt and for taking a chance on a first-time author who said 'fuck' too much.

I also said 'ugh' too much, which was pointed out by my kind and talented editors Abigail Le Marquand-Brown and Kate Fox. They both remained patient and helpful throughout the process of shaping this waffly rant of my consciousness into a book, and even said some of my jokes were funny. Some. Not all. Thank you, Abi and Kate, for your helpful commentary and your patience with the PDF/Google Doc hellfests and my occasional (ahem) angry feminist agenda. HQ at HarperCollins is consistently publishing bold books from clever women, and I'm thrilled that I managed to sneak into their roster.

Thanks also to my therapist, Marcelle Casingena, who didn't once tell me to get a grip as I sat blubbering and snotting in front of her in a strange, grey room in North London. Marcelle's kindness, patience and clever therapist-wizard-techniques helped me become kinder to myself, and to vanquish a fair amount of the depression demons who were circling.

Overly affectionate thanks have to go to my non-qualified therapist, Tom Miller, who has been the Thelma to my Louise and the Beverley to my Karen for far too many years than we'd each like to admit. Tom is there for me when I have middle-of-the-night-freak-outs, middle-of-the-day-sobs and middle-part-of-life-wrinkle-crises, and has been there for me without realizing how much he's been there and how much his kind yet cynical presence means to me. Also, he makes a filthy Nigella pasta. Love you hunty.

Thanks to Dré for keeping me in Yazoo and cuddles for sixteen cherished years, and for being OK with me writing about quite personal parts of our relationship for a mass audience of maybe up to six people.

If you are one of those six people reading this (including the ever-supportive Bin Sick WhatsApp group – thanks for reassuring me all the damn time), then of course, thank you to you, too. I hope that there was one line or paragraph of my witterings that helped you or could help someone close to you. When you're in the middle of the darkest times, it seems like nothing will put out your brain fires and that they're all your fault. I hope this book has made you see that they're not your fault at all, and that although the fire might not completely go out, it will one day just be burning embers.

If you thought the whole thing was crap then I guess that's fine, too, but don't make a public declaration of it, yeah?

xx

ONE PLACE. MANY STORIES

Bold, innovative and
empowering publishing.

FOLLOW US ON:

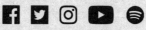

@HQStories